主 编 顾建钧 郁东海

执行主编 娄继权 何文忠 乔 韵

针灸推拿

实践操作指导

（汉英对照）

GUIDE ON THE PRACTICE OF ACUPUNCTURE, MOXIBUSTION AND TUINA

(Chinese-English Version)

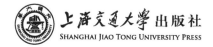

上海交通大学出版社
SHANGHAI JIAO TONG UNIVERSITY PRESS

内容提要

　　本书分为三大部分,第一部分简要介绍中医基础理论知识;第二部分主要为推拿实践操作;第三部分主要介绍针灸实践操作。本书在内容上注重实践操作、英文翻译选词浅显易懂,重在交流方便。本书为中英文对照教材,既可以作为中医药国际化人才培训班的培训教材,提高中医药人才的专业英语水平;同时因为内容具有实用性,选词浅显易懂,也能够作为外籍医务人员中医培训的参考书目,以传播中医医学知识,更好地推动中医药国际化。

图书在版编目(CIP)数据

针灸推拿实践操作指导: 汉英对照/顾建钧,郁东海主编.
—上海:上海交通大学出版社,2017
ISBN 978 - 7 - 313 - 17428 - 4

Ⅰ.①针… Ⅱ.①顾…②郁… Ⅲ.①针灸学—汉、英
②推拿—汉、英 Ⅳ.①R24

中国版本图书馆 CIP 数据核字(2017)第 147282 号

针灸推拿实践操作指导(汉英对照)

主　　　编:	顾建钧　郁东海			
出版发行:	上海交通大学出版社		地　　址:	上海市番禺路 951 号
邮政编码:	200030		电　　话:	021-64071208
出 版 人:	郑益慧			
印　　制:	上海天地海设计印刷有限公司		经　　销:	全国新华书店
开　　本:	787mm×1092mm　1/16		印　　张:	12.25
字　　数:	270 千字			
版　　次:	2017 年 6 月第 1 版		印　　次:	2017 年 6 月第 1 次印刷
书　　号:	ISBN 978 - 7 - 313 - 17428 - 4/R			
定　　价:	58.00 元			

编委会名单

主　　编　顾建钧　郁东海

执行主编　娄继权　何文忠　乔　韵

副 主 编　孙　敏　骆智琴　兰　蕾

主　　审　李征宇　关　鑫

编　　委　(按姓氏笔画顺序排列)

马辰吟　卞亚琴　叶　盛　冯　旻

庄悦红　朱　俊　杨燕婷　何腾飞

吴玥凡　晋　永　贾文鹏　谢洁静

前　言
Preface

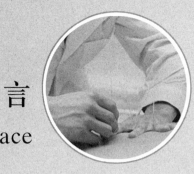

　　中医药学是中国的传统医学科学。它拥有内科、外科、针灸、推拿、骨伤、肛肠等不同的治疗领域，为炎黄子孙的健康做出了不可磨灭的贡献。从 20 世纪 70 年代开始，中医针灸开始走出国门，在国外产生了"针灸热潮"，甚至有美国西医专家团组团来中国感受针灸的神奇魅力。至今为止，中医的针灸推拿技术已走出国门，走向世界，其疗效之显著在国际上产生了巨大的轰动。现在在美国、英国、加拿大、日本、韩国、泰国等多个国家都有专门的中医学院，每年也有大批留学生赴中国学习中医。

　　同时，党和政府也高度重视中医药国际化，2015 年 6 月 22 日，捷克赫拉德茨 - 克拉洛维州立医院中医中心正式成立，这是中东欧地区首家由两国政府支持的中医机构。2016 年 2 月 22 日国务院出台的《关于印发中医药发展战略规划纲要（2016—2030 年）》，强调"加强中医药对外交流合作"。为了做好中医药对外交流合作的工作，培养一批具有国际交流能力的复合型中医药人才势在必行。浦东新区作为国家中医药发展综合改革试验区，也高度重视中医药复合型人才的培养。因此，2016 年 3 月，在浦东新区国际医学交流中心的牵头下，首届国际化复合型中医药人才培训班开班。

　　为了使培训规范化、体系化，有长足的发展机制，我们根据实践经验，并参照中医基础理论、针灸和推拿教材、诊疗规范要求，针对国内中医医务人员出国常用的中医诊疗技术，组织编撰了《针灸推拿实践操作指导》（*Guide on the Practice of Acupunture，Moxibustion and Tuina*）。该教材的编写原则是内容上注重实践操作，英文翻译选词浅显易懂，重在交流方便。因此，该教材既可以作为中医药国际化人才培训班的培训教材，提高中医药人才的专业英语水平；同时因为内容具有实用性，选词浅显易懂，也能够作为外籍医务人员中医培训的参考书目，以传播中医医学知识，更好地推动中医药国际化。

在编写过程中，我们邀请了针灸、推拿领域的权威专家进行审稿和校对，力求做到准确、简洁、明了、实用。由于时间紧迫，编辑过程中存在的疏漏，望同道和读者不吝赐教。

本书在编写过程中，得到了浦东新区卫生和计划生育委员会、上海中医药大学相关领导的指导和支持，全体编写人员在此表示由衷地感谢。

编　者

2017 年 3 月

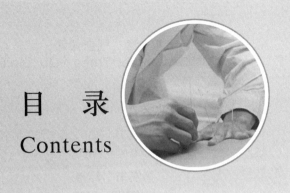

目　录
Contents

第二部分　推　拿
Part Two　Tuina

第三部分　针灸和其他
Part Three　Acupuncture and Moxibustion and the Other

第一部分
中医基础理论
Part One   Basic Theory of Traditional Chinese Medicine

中医学是中国人民长期同疾病做斗争的经验总结,是我国优秀文化的一个重要组成部分。通过长期的医疗实践,它逐步形成并发展成为独特的医学理论体系,为中国人民的健康做出了巨大的贡献。

　　Traditional Chinese Medicine (TCM) is a summary on the Chinese people's experience in fighting against diseases and also an essential part of Chinese culture. Through generations of medical practice, it has evolved into an unique medical theoretical system, making huge contributions to the health of Chinese people.

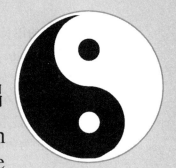

第一章 中医学哲学基础

Chapter One Philosophical Foundation of Traditional Chinese Medicine

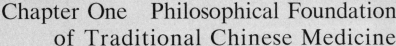

第一节 阴阳学说

Section One The Theory of Yin and Yang

一、阴阳的基本概念

阴阳是对自然界相互关联的某些事物和现象对立双方属性的概括。阴阳学说是研究事物阴阳的属性及其运动变化规律,并用以阐释宇宙万物的发生、发展和变化的古代哲学思想,是古代朴素的宇宙观和方法论。

Ⅰ. Basic Concept of Yin and Yang

Yin and yang represent two opposite but complementary qualities of interrelated things or phenomena in the natural world. With focus on the attributes, movements and changes of each quality, the theory of yin and yang can be used to illustrate the emergence, development and changes of every being in the universe. Therefore, it can be regarded as the view of the universe and methodology in ancient times.

二、阴阳学说的基本内容

1. 阴阳对立制约

阴阳相反,导致阴阳相互制约。阴阳双方制约的结果,使事物取得了动态平衡。

2. 阴阳互根互用

阴阳互根是指一切事物或现象中相互对立着的阴阳两个方面,具有相互依存、互为根本的关系,即阴和阳任何一方都不能脱离另一方面而单独存在。阳依存于阴,阴依存于阳。这种相互依存关系,称之为"互根"。"互用"是指阴阳双方不断地滋生、促进和助长对方。

3．阴阳的消长平衡

消，即减少；长，即增加。阴阳消长是指一事物中所含阴阳的量和阴与阳之间的比例不是一成不变的，而是不断地消长变化着。

4．阴阳的相互转化

阴阳转化，是指一事物总体属性在一定条件下，可以向其相反的方向转化，即阳的事物可发展转化为阴的事物，而阴的事物也可以转化为属阳的事物。

Ⅱ．Basic Content of the Theory of Yin and Yang

1．The Opposition of Yin and Yang

Yin and yang are mutually opposed to each other, which leads to mutual restriction of two parts, promoting dynamic balance.

2．Interdependence and Promotion of Yin and Yang

Although yin and yang are opposite, they are interdependent. One cannot exist without the other. Yang depends on yin and yin depends on yang too. This is what we call interdependence. Besides, promotion of yin and yang means that yin can foster yang, and *vice versa*.

3．Waning and Waxing Between Yin and Yang

Waning means decrease and waxing means increasing. Yin and yang coexist in a dynamic balance in which one waxes while the other wanes. In other words, yin and yang are constantly changing and not static.

4．Inter-transformation of Yin and Yang

Under some circumstances, either yin or yang may transform into its opposite side. In other words, yang can transform into yin and *vice versa*.

三、阴阳学说在中医学中的应用

阴阳学说，贯穿在中医学理论体系的各个方面，用来说明人体的组织结构、生理功能、疾病的发生发展规律，并指导着临床诊断和治疗。

Ⅲ．Application of the Theory in TCM

The theory of yin and yang is reflected in every aspect of TCM theoretical system. For example, it can be used for explaining the structure of human body, physiological functions, the development of diseases and also for guiding clinical diagnosis and treatment.

第二节 五行学说
Section Two The Theory of Five Elements

一、五行的基本概念和特性

1. 概念
五行指木、火、土、金、水五种物质及其运动变化。

2. 五行各自的特性
（1）木的特性：生长、柔和、曲直。

（2）火的特性：温热、上升。

（3）土的特性：生化、承载、受纳。

（4）金的特性：沉降、肃杀、收敛。

（5）水的特性：滋润、下行、寒凉、闭藏。

Ⅰ. Basic Concept and Qualities

1. Basic Concept
Five elements refer to five substances, namely wood, fire, earth, metal and water, and the movements and changes of them.

2. Qualities of Each Element
（1）Wood is characterized by growing freely, ascending and developing freely. It can be bent and straightened.

（2）Fire is featured by warming and rising.

（3）Earth is characterized by generating, transforming, supporting and receiving.

（4）Metal is featured by purifying, descending and astringing.

（5）Water is characterized by moistening, downward flowing, cooling and storing.

二、五行生克和乘侮

1. 五行的相生
（1）含义：木、火、土、金、水之间存在着有序的依次滋生、助长和促进关系。

（2）相生顺序：木→火→土→金→水→木。

2. 五行的相克
（1）含义：木、火、土、金、水之间存在依次克制、制约的关系。

（2）相克顺序：木（克）→土（克）→水（克）→火（克）→金（克）→木。

3. 五行的相乘
含义：指五行中某"一行"对被克的"一行"克制太过，从而引起一系列异常相克的反应。

4. 五行的相侮

含义：指五行中的某"一行"过于强盛，对原来"克我"的"一行"进行反侮。

Ⅱ. The Generation, Restriction, Over-restriction and Counter-restriction of Five Elements

1. Generation

(1) Definition: Generation of five elements means that each element engenders and promotes another sequential element.

(2) Sequence: wood→fire→earth→metal→water→wood.

2. Restriction

(1) Definition: Restriction of five elements means that each element restricts and controls another sequential element.

(2) Sequence: wood→earth→water→fire→metal→wood.

3. Over-restriction

Definition: Over-restriction refers to an abnormal condition in which one element of the five elements excessively restricts its restricting element.

4. Counter-restriction

Definition: Counter-restriction means the reverse restraint. In this abnormal condition, one element is over-predominant and reversely restrains and bullies the element that restricts it.

三、五行学说在中医学中的应用

五行学说在中医学中的应用，主要是以五行的特性来分析研究脏腑经络等的五行属性；以生克来分析脏腑、经络之间和各个生理功能之间的相互关系；以乘侮来阐释病理情况下的相互影响。

Ⅲ. Application of the Theory in TCM

The theory of five elements is mainly used for analyzing the attribution of five elements in zang-fu organs, meridians and collaterals by their features, to analyze and study the mutual relationships in the zang-fu organs, meridians and in various physiological functions by the generating and restricting relationships among the five elements, and to explain the mutual influence in the pathological conditions by the over-restricting and counter-restricting relationships of the five elements.

第三节　中医学理论体系的主要特点
Section Three　Characteristics of Traditional Chinese Medicine Theoretical System

一、整体观念

人体是一个有机的整体,人与自然界和社会息息相关、密切相连;同时,在人体内部,人体结构组织和功能也具有整体性。这两大方面共同构成了中医理论的整体观念。

Ⅰ. The Holism

Human being is an organic whole, which is closely related with the nature and the society they live in. In addition, in a body, the structure and the function of each part are integrated whole. These are the two parts of the holism.

二、辨证论治

辨证论治包括辨证和论治两方面,是中医察识和治疗疾病的基本法则。辨证包括三个步骤,就是通过对四诊(望、闻、问、切)所收集的临床资料(包括症状、体征、病史)进行分析、归纳和综合,从而辨识出疾病在这一特定时间范围的原因、病位、性质及邪正关系等病理本质内容,并归纳为某一证。

论治,则是在辨证基础上所确定的治疗法则。

Ⅱ. Treatment Based on Pattern Identification

Treatment based on pattern identification includes two parts, namely pattern identification and treatment. It is the basic principle for diagnosing and treating diseases with TCM. Pattern identification involves three steps: to make a comprehensive analysis on the clinical data collected through four diagnostic methods (inspection, auscultation and olfaction, inquiry and palpation), to draw a diagnostic conclusion on the current conditions like etiology, disease location, disease nature, and the struggle between body resistance and pathological factors, and to summarize a pattern.

Treatment refers to the therapeutic principle determined by the pattern which is identified before.

第二章 藏 象
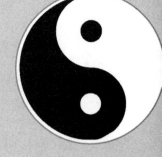

Chapter Two　Visceral Manifestations

藏象学说是以脏腑为基础。按照脏腑的生理功能特点,可分为五脏、六腑和奇恒之腑。

The theory of visceral manifestations is based on zang-fu organs. According to the physiological functions, organs can be divided into three categories, namely five zang-organs, six fu-organs and extraordinary organs.

第一节　五　脏
Section One　Five Zang-organs

五脏指的是心、肝、脾、肺、肾。其共同的生理功能是化生和贮藏精气。

Five zang-organs refer to the heart, the liver, the spleen, the lungs and the kidneys. They share a common physiological function, to transform and store essence.

一、心

1. 生理功能

(1) 心主血脉。①心行血,即心气推动和调控血液在脉中正常运行,使其流注全身,以输送营养物质、滋润和濡养各脏腑五体官窍。②心生血,即心火(心阳)能将进入心脉的营气和津液化赤为血。

(2) 心藏神:①统帅全身脏腑、经络、五体、官窍的生理活动;②主司意识、思维、情志等精神活动。人的意识、思维、情志等精神活动,是脏腑精气对外界环境刺激而做出应答反应的结果;是在心神的主导下,由五脏协作、共同来完成的。

2. 特点

在体合脉,其华在面,在窍为舌,在志为喜,在液为汗,与夏气相通应。

Ⅰ. The heart

1. Physiological Functions

(1) The heart is in charge of blood and vessels: ① The heart promotes blood circulation. Heart qi propels and regulates the blood circulation, distributing blood and nutrients to the body so as to moisten and nourish zang-fu organs, five body constituents and orifices. ②The heart generates blood. Heart fire (heart yang) can transform the nutrient qi and fluids that are carried into the heart to the blood.

(2) The heart stores shen (spirit or mind): ① The heart dominates the physiological activities of zang-fu organs, meridians and collaterals, five body constituents and orifices. ② The heart controls mental activities, such as consciousness, thinking and emotions. Dominated by heart shen, all these activities are the responses of zang-fu organs and essences to the outside world.

2. Characteristics

The heart corresponds to vessels and opens into the tongue, manifesting on the face, associating with joy in emotions, sweat in fluids, being harmony with the qi of summer.

二、肝

1. 生理功能

(1) 肝主疏泄：是指肝气具有疏通、畅达全身气机，进而促进精血津液的运行输布、脾胃之气的升降、胆汁的分泌排泄以及情志的舒畅等作用。维持全身脏腑、经络、五体、官窍功能活动稳定有序。

(2) 肝藏血：是指肝脏具有贮藏血液、调节血量和防止出血的功能。

2. 特点

在体合筋，其华在爪，在窍为目，在志为怒，在液为泪，与春气相通应。

Ⅱ. The Liver

1. Physiological Functions

(1) The liver governs soothing. This means that liver qi can promote the free flow of qi, thereby propelling the distribution and transportation of essence, blood and fluids, the ascending and descending of spleen qi and stomach qi, secretion and distribution of bile and emotions. Therefore, zang-fu organs, meridians and collaterals, five body constituents and orifices can function properly.

(2) The liver stores blood. It means the liver can house and regulate blood, and prevent bleeding.

2．Characteristics

The liver corresponds to sinews and opens into the eyes, manifesting on the nails, associating with anger in emotions, tear in fluids, being harmony with the qi of spring.

三、脾

1．生理功能

（1）脾主运化：是指脾具有把饮食水谷转化为水谷精微和津液，并把水谷精微和津液吸收、转输到全身各脏腑的生理功能，故称为"后天之本"。

（2）脾主统血：是指脾气具有统摄、控制血液在脉中正常运行而不逸出脉外的功能。

2．特点

在体合肉，主四肢，在窍为口，其华在唇，在志为思，在液为涎，与长夏之气相通应。

Ⅲ．The spleen

1．Physiological Functions

（1）The spleen governs transportation and transformation. It means that the spleen can transform the water and cereals into cereal essence and fluids, and then absorb and distribute them into every organs of the body. Therefore, it is called the root of acquired constitution.

（2）The spleen commands blood, which means that spleen qi can keep the blood circulating within the vessels and prevent bleeding.

2．Characteristics

The spleen controls the muscles and four limbs, and opens into the mouth, manifesting on lips, associating with pensiveness in emotions, saliva in fluids, being harmony with the qi of long summer.

四、肺

1．生理功能

（1）主气（司呼吸）：肺主气，包括主呼吸之气和主一身之气两个方面。①肺主呼吸之气，是指肺主管呼吸，是体内外气体交换的场所。②肺主一身之气，是指肺有主司一身之气的生成和运行的作用，对全身气机的调节作用。

（2）主行水：是指肺气的宣发肃降作用推动和调节全身水液的输布和排泄。

（3）肺朝百脉：是指全身的血液都通过百脉流经于肺，经肺的呼吸，进行体内外清浊之气的交换；然后再通过肺气宣降作用，将富有清气的血液通过百脉输送到全身。

（4）肺主治节：是指肺气具有治理调节肺之呼吸及全身之气、血、水的作用。

2．特点

在体合皮，其华在毛，在窍为鼻，在志为忧（悲），在液为涕，与秋气相通应。

Ⅳ. The Lungs

1. Physiological Functions

(1) The lungs control qi and respiration. It has two meanings. On the one hand, the lungs control the qi that is inhaled in and exhaled out, for they are the places where the qi in the body exchanges with the fresh air. On the other hand, the lungs dominate the qi of the body, for it can promote the generation and circulation of the qi and regulate the qi movement.

(2) The lungs promote water movement. Lung qi regulates the distribution and discharge of water by diffusing and descending.

(3) The lungs govern hundreds of vessels. It means that the blood circulates into the lungs via vessels and then exchanges with the fresh air by respiration. By diffusing and descending, lung qi distributes the blood rich in fresh air to the whole body via vessels.

(4) The lungs govern management and regulation. Lung qi manages respiration and regulates the distribution of qi, blood and water in the whole body.

2. Characteristics

The lungs correspond to skin and open into the nose, manifesting on body hair, associating with sorrow and grief in emotions, snivel in fluids, being harmony with the qi of autumn.

五、肾

1. 生理功能

（1）肾藏精：是指肾具有贮藏精气的生理功能。精，是构成人体和维持人体生命活动的最基本物质，是脏腑、五体、官窍功能活动的物质基础，主生长、发育、生殖与脏腑气化。人体生命过程中的每一阶段机体的生长发育或衰退情况，都取决于肾精及肾气的盛衰。

（2）肾主水：是指肾气具有主司和调节全身水液代谢的功能。

（3）肾主纳气：是指肾气有摄纳肺所吸入的自然界清气，保持吸气的深度，防止呼吸表浅的作用。

2. 特点

在体合骨、生髓，其华在发，在窍为耳及二阴，在志为恐，在液为唾，与冬气相通应。

Ⅴ. The Kidneys

1. Physiological Functions

(1) The kidneys store essence. Essence is a fundamental substance for body and life activities and also a basic substance for zang-fu organs, five body constituents and

orifices to function properly. Therefore, the kidneys govern growth, development, reproduction and qi transformation as well. In a conclusion, every stage of human life, growth, development or even aging, all depends on the waxing and waning of kidney essence and kidney qi.

（2）The kidneys dominate water, which means that kidney qi can command and regulate water metabolism.

（3）The kidneys control qi-receiving. It refers to the kidney qi receiving fresh air inhaled by the lungs and holding it down. Thus, breathlessness can be prevented.

2．Characteristics

The kidneys correspond to bones, generate marrow and open into the ears and two lower orifices, manifesting on hair, associating with fright in emotions, spittle in fluids, being harmony with the qi of winter.

第二节 六 腑
Section Two   Six Fu-organs

六腑指的是胆、胃、小肠、大肠、膀胱、三焦。其共同的生理功能是受盛和传化水谷。

Six fu-organs refer to the gallbladder, the stomach, the small intestine, the large intestine, the bladder and the triple energizers. They share a common physiological function, to receive, transport and transform water and food.

一、胆

胆贮藏和排泄胆汁。胆汁来源于肝之余气，由肝血化生。在肝气疏泄功能的作用下分泌胆汁，进入胆腑浓缩、贮藏；随着消化过程的需要，在肝胆之气疏泄功能的共同作用下，贮藏于胆腑的胆汁通过输胆管排泄而注入肠中，以促进食物的消化和吸收。

Ⅰ．The Gallbladder

The gallbladder stores and excretes bile. Bile stems from the extra liver qi and is transformed by liver blood. With the soothing function of liver qi, bile is excreted and then condensed and stored in the gallbladder. When needed in digestion, affected by soothing function, the stored bile is discharged via bile duct and then enters intestines to aid digestion and absorption.

二、胃

胃主受纳水谷，腐熟水谷。胃气具有接受和容纳饮食物的作用，因此胃有"太仓""水谷之海""水谷气血之海"之称。同时,胃气还可以将食物初步消化,并形成食糜。胃气的两个功能必须与脾气的运化功能相互配合,纳运协调才能将水谷化为精微,进而化生精气血津液,供养全身。

Ⅱ . The Stomach

The stomach controls receiving, rotting and ripening food. As stomach qi receives food, the stomach is also regarded as "great granary" "the sea of food and drink" or "the sea of food and drink, qi and blood". In the meantime, stomach qi digests the food into chyme. However, to properly transform food into essence, stomach qi must cooperate with spleen qi in transportation and transformation. Furthermore, essence, qi, blood and fluids can be generated to nourish the whole body.

三、小肠

小肠主受盛化物,泌别清浊。受盛化物是指小肠接受胃腑下传的食糜,并对其进一步消化和吸收精微的功能。泌别清浊是指小肠将经过消化的食糜,分为精微(包括水分)和残渣两部分,吸收精微物质和水分,把食物残渣下送大肠的作用。由于小肠在吸收水谷精微的同时,还吸收了大量的水液,参与了人体的水液代谢,所以有"小肠主液"的说法。

Ⅲ . The Small Intestine

The small intestine governs receiving, transforming and separating the turbid from the clear. After receiving the chyme passed down from the stomach, the small intestine further digests it and absorbs the essence. After absorption, the small intestine separates the chyme into essence (including fluids) and remainings, and passes down the remainings into the large intestine. In the meantime, the small intestine absorbs the essence and fluids as well. Therefore, it is involved into water metabolism. That's why we've got a saying that the small intestine controls the fluids.

四、大肠

大肠主传化糟粕。大肠接受经过小肠泌别清浊后剩余的食物残渣与水液,吸收其中多余的水分,形成粪便,传送至大肠的末端,经肛门有节制地排出体外。大肠在接受小肠下注的食物残渣,再吸收其中剩余的水分,在一定程度上影响水液的代谢,故称"大肠主津"。

Ⅳ . The Large Intestine

The large intestine controls passage and conduction. After receiving the remainings passed down from the small intestine, the large intestine continues to absorb the liquids and transforms the rest into stools simultaneously. Finally, the stools are passed down into the anus and discharged. Because of the liquid reabsorption, the large intestine is involved into water metabolism. Therefore, the large intestine controls the liquids.

五、膀胱

膀胱主贮存和排泄尿液，其功能依赖于肾气与膀胱之气的升降协调。

Ⅴ. The Bladder

The bladder stores and discharges urine, which relies on the ascending and descending of kidney qi and bladder qi.

六、三焦

三焦主运行元气、水谷与水液。

Ⅵ. Triple Energizers

Ttriple energizer governs the movement of origin qi, food and water.

第三节　奇恒之腑
Section Three　Extraordinary Organs

奇恒之腑指形态上中空有腔似腑，功能上贮藏精气似脏的脏腑。

Extraordinary organs refer to those hollow organs with functions of storing essence.

一、脑

（1）脑为元神之府，能主宰人体的生命活动。

（2）脑主人的意识、思维、记忆、情志等精神活动。

（3）司感觉。眼、耳、口、鼻、舌等五脏外窍，皆位于头面，与脑相通。人的视觉、听觉、味觉、嗅觉等感觉，皆与脑有密切关系。

Ⅰ. The Brain

（1）As a house for original shen，the brain controls life activities.

（2）It governs consciousness, thinking, memory and emotions.

（3）It controls senses and sports. As the external orifices of five zang-organs, eyes, ears, mouth, nose and tongue are situated on the face and connected with the brain. Therefore, the brain is closely related to sight, hearing, smell and taste.

二、女子胞

女子胞主持月经,胞宫的形态与功能正常与否直接影响月经的来潮。同时女子胞是孕育胎儿的器官。

Ⅱ. The Uterus

The uterus regulates menstruation. Its form and function can influence the menstruation. Meanwhile, the uterus houses the fetus during pregnancy.

第四节　脏与脏的关系
Section Four   The Relationship Between Zang-organs and Zang-organs

一、心与肺

心主一身之血,心气推动血行,是肺朝百脉的基础;肺主一身之气,肺气能够辅助心气推动血行。心肺两脏相互协调,保证了气血的正常运行,维持着各脏腑组织器官的新陈代谢。主要表现在血液运行和呼吸吐纳之间的协同调节关系。

Ⅰ. The Heart and the Lungs

The heart governs the blood and heart qi is responsible for propelling blood circulation, which is the foundation for the lungs to carry blood with qi to circulate around the body. The lungs governs the qi and lung qi can assist heart qi to promote blood circulation. Therefore, the cooperation between the heart and the lungs guarantees the normal circulation of qi and blood, maintain the metabolism of other organs. In a conclusion, the relationship between two zang-organs is reflected in two aspects: blood circulation and respiration.

二、心与脾

心主一身之血,心气推动血行,供养脾脏,脾得滋养则能健运,化生血液的功能也就旺盛;脾主运化,化生水谷精微,并将水谷精微上输于心肺,化生为血。因此,脾气健运,则血液化生有源,以保证心血充盈。

血液在脉中正常运行,既有赖于心气的推动,以维持通畅而不迟缓、瘀滞,又依靠脾气的统摄,以保证血行脉中而不逸出脉外。

主要表现在血液生成方面的相互为用和血液运行方面的相互协同。

Ⅱ. The Heart and the Spleen

The heart governs blood and heart qi propels blood to circulate around the body, especially the spleen. Therefore, the spleen gets nourished and is able to transport and to generate blood. As the spleen is in charge of transforming water and grains into essence and transporting them to the heart and the lung where the essence is transformed into blood. Therefore, with the transporting functions of spleen qi, the blood gets its source so that the heart blood is guaranteed.

The circulation of blood depends on the propelling of heart qi and also the controlling of spleen qi. The heart qi promotes smooth blood circulation and the spleen qi controls the blood in the vessels.

In a conclusion, the relationship between two zang-organs is reflected in two aspects: blood generation and circulation.

三、心与肝

心血充盈、心气旺盛，则血行正常、肝有所藏；肝血充足、肝气疏泄有度，能随人体生理需求进行血量调节，也有利于心行血功能的正常运行。

心血充盈、心神健旺，有助于肝气疏泄、情志调畅；而肝气疏泄有度，则情志畅快。所以，心肝两脏相互为用，共同维持正常的精神活动。

主要表现在行血、藏血和精神调节三个方面。

Ⅲ. The Heart and the Liver

With sufficient heart blood and heart qi, the blood can circulate around and be stored in the liver. When the liver stores ample blood, the liver qi can soothe properly and regulate the blood volume according to the physiological needs of the body, which is also beneficial to the blood circulation.

Ample blood and vital spirit are conducive to soothing liver qi and regulating emotions. Therefore, the heart and the liver can work together to maintain normal mental activities.

In a conclusion, the relationship between these two zang-organs is mirrored in three aspects: blood circulating, blood storing and emotion regulating.

四、心与肾

主要表现为"心肾相交"。其机制，主要从以下三个方面来阐述。

1. 水火既济

心火必须下降于肾,使肾水不寒;肾水必须上济于心,使心火不亢。通过心与肾之间的水火升降互济,维持了两脏之间生理功能的协调平衡。

2. 精神互用

心藏神,肾藏精。精能化气生神,为气、神之源;神能控精驭气,为精、气之主。

3. 君相安位

心为君火,为一身之主宰;肾为相火,系阳气之根,为神明之基础。心阳与肾阳可相互资助。君火相火,各安其位,则心肾上下交济。主要表现为"心肾相交"。

IV. The Heart and the Kidneys

The relationship between the heart and the kidneys is mainly shown in the interaction between these two organs. It can be illustrated in the following three aspects.

1. The Interaction Between Fire and Water

The heart fire needs to descend down to the kidneys to make sure the warmth of kidney water, while kidney water must ascend to the heart to prevent the exuberance of heart fire. Through the interaction between these two organs, the physiological functions between the two organs can be balanced.

2. The Essence and Spirit Benefiting Each Other

The heart stores spirit, while the kidneys store essence. Essence is the source of qi and spirit, for it can be transformed into qi and be generated into spirit. The spirit is the master of essence and qi, for it can control the qi.

3. Sovereign and Minister Adhering to Their Own Duties

The heart is sovereign fire which controls the whole body, while the kidneys are also called minister fire, the root of yang qi and also the basis of spirit. Heart yang and kidney yang can assist each other. They can also adhere to their own duties, thus promoting the upward and downward interaction.

五、肺与脾

主要体现在气的生成和水液代谢两个方面。

1. 气的生成方面

在气的生成方面:肺吸入的自然界清气和脾化生水谷之精所化的谷气,在肺中相结合而生成宗气。脾所化生的谷精、谷气与津液有赖于肺气的宣降运动而输布全身。而肺维持其生理活动所需要的谷精、谷气与津液,又依靠脾气运化水谷的作用生成。

2. 水液代谢方面

在水液代谢方面:肺气宣降以行水,有助于脾的运化水液功能;而脾气运化水液,散精于肺,又是肺主行水的前提。所以,肺脾两脏协调配合,相互为用,是保证津液正常输布与排泄的重要环节。

Ⅴ. The Lungs and the Spleen

The relationship between the lungs and the spleen is reflected in two parts: the generation of qi and water metabolism.

1. In Terms of Qi Generation

In terms of qi Generation, in the lungs, the fresh air inhaled from the nature is combined with the cereal qi transformed from water and grains by the spleen, thus pectoral qi is generated. The distribution of cereal essence, cereal qi and fluids transformed by the spleen relies on the dispersing and descending of lung qi, while in order to maintain its own physiological functions, the lungs also need cereal essence, cereal qi and fluids which are transformed from water and grains by the spleen qi.

2. In Terms of Water Metabolism

As for water metabolism, lung qi disperses and descends, which is conducive to transporting and transforming water. In return, spleen qi transports water and disperses essence to the lungs, which is the precondition for the lungs to move water. Therefore, the cooperation of the lungs and the spleen is an essential link for the normal distribution and discharge of fluids and liquids.

六、肺与肝

主要体现在人体气机升降的调节方面。肝气疏泄、升发条达,有利于肺气的肃降;肺气充足、肃降正常,又有利于肝气的升发。两者协调平衡,对全身气机的调畅、气血的调和,起着重要的调节作用。

Ⅵ. The Lungs and the Liver

The relationship between the lungs and the liver is mainly represented in the regulation of qi movement. The liver soothes qi and governs ascending and dispersing, which is beneficial to the descending of lung qi. In return, sufficient lung qi and normal descending can promote the soothing of liver qi. A balance between them will play a key role in regulating the qi movement within the whole body and also in harmonizing the qi and blood.

七、肺与肾

主要体现在水液代谢和呼吸运动两个方面。

1. 水液代谢方面

肺气宣肃而行水的功能,有赖于肾气及肾阴肾阳的促进;肾气所蒸化及升降的水液,也有赖于肺气的肃降作用使之下归于肾或膀胱。肺肾之气的协同作用,保证了体内水液输布与排泄的正常。

2. 呼吸运动方面

在人体呼吸运动中,肺气肃降,有利于肾的纳气;肾精肾气充足、摄纳有力,也有利于肺气的肃降。

Ⅶ. The Lungs and the Kidneys

The relationship between these two zang-organs can be reflected into two aspects: water metabolism and respiration.

1. In Terms of Water Metabolism

On one hand, lung qi moves water by dispersing and descending. This function relies on the kidney qi, kidney yin and kidney yang. On the other hand, Kidney qi steams, ascends and descends water. To work properly, lung qi needs to descend to the kidneys or the bladder. The collaboration of lung qi and kidney qi guarantees the normal distribution and discharge of water.

2. In Terms of Respiration

As for respiration, lung qi descends, which helps the kidneys to receive qi. Sufficient kidney essence and kidney qi can also boost the descending of lung qi.

八、肝与脾

主要体现在饮食物消化、血液运行两大方面。

1. 饮食物消化方面

肝主疏泄,调畅气机,通过协调脾胃升降和促进胆汁的分泌、排泄,能够助脾运化。脾胃的升降为一身气机升降的枢纽;而且脾气健运,水谷精微化生充足,气血生化有源,肝体得养而使肝气冲和条达。

2. 血液运行方面

脾气健旺、生血有源、统血有权,使肝有所藏而能正常调节血量;肝血充足、藏泻有度,血容量得以正常调节,使脾的生理活动能得到足够的血液供养。所以,肝脾相互协作,共同维持血液的正常运行。

Ⅷ. The Liver and the Spleen

The relationship between these two zang-organs can be mirrored into two aspects: food digestion and blood circulation.

1. In Terms of Food Digestion

The liver regulates the flow of qi and thus promote the ascending and descending of the spleen and the stomach, and bile excretion and discharge. In this way, the liver can aid the spleen in transportation and transformation. In addition, the spleen and the stomach are the hubs of qi movement. If spleen qi is vigorous, cereal essence will be abundant for the generation of qi and blood. Thus, the liver will get nourished and liver qi will flow smoothly.

2. In Terms of Blood Circulation

As for blood circulation, with vigorous spleen qi, the blood has got enough sources and the spleen can command blood. Therefore, the liver has enough blood storage and thus can regulate the blood volume. With adequate liver blood, the liver can regulate the blood volume by storing and discharging when needed. In this way, the spleen is nourished so that it can function properly. Therefore, the liver and the spleen cooperate to maintain the generation and circulation of blood.

九、肝与肾

主要表现在精血同源、藏泄互用以及阴阳互滋互制等三个方面。

1. 精血同源方面

肾精和肝血之间存在着相互滋生和相互转化的关系，而且精和血皆由水谷之精化生和充养，故称之为"精血同源互化"。

2. 藏泄互用方面

肝气疏泄与肾气封藏，相反而相成，从而调节女子的月经来潮、排卵和男子的排精功能。

3. 阴阳互滋互制方面

肾阴滋养肝阴，共同制约肝阳，则肝阳不偏亢；肾阳资助肝阳，共同温煦肝脉，可防止肝脉寒滞。

Ⅸ. The Liver and the Kidneys

The relationship between these two zang-organs can be shown into three parts: essence and blood sharing a common source, coordination of storing and discharging, and mutual nourishment and mutual restriction of yin and yang.

1. Essence and Blood Sharing a Common Source

As for essence and blood sharing a common source, kidney essence and liver blood can generate and transform to each other. Besides, both essence and blood stem from cereal essence. Therefore, it is believed that the essence shares a common source with blood.

2. Coordination of Storing and Discharging

In terms of storing and discharging, liver qi soothes and kidney qi stores. Due to the opposition, they can restrict and coordinate with each other, thereby regulating menstruation, ovulation and spermiation.

3. Mutual Nourishment and Mutual Restriction of Yin and Yang

As for mutual nourishment and mutual restriction of yin and yang, Kidney yin nourishes liver yin and restricts liver yang together with liver yin, so liver yang won't be exuberant. In addition, kidney yang aids liver yang, and both of them warm the liver vessels to prevent the cold coagulation.

十、脾与肾

主要体现在先天与后天互促互助及水液代谢两个方面。

1. 先天与后天方面

在先天与后天相互滋生、相互促进方面,脾运化水谷的功能,有赖于肾气及肾阴肾阳的资助和促进,才能健旺,即所谓"先天温养、激发后天";肾所藏先天之精及其化生的元气,也有赖于脾气运化的水谷之精及其化生的谷气的不断充养和培育,才能充盛,即所谓"后天补充、培育先天"。

2. 水液代谢方面

在协同维持水液代谢的协调平衡方面,脾气运化水液功能的正常发挥,必须依赖肾气的蒸化及肾阳的温煦作用的支持。肾气主司水液代谢,又必须依赖脾气及脾阳的协助。脾肾两脏相互协同,共同主司水液代谢的协调平衡。

Ⅹ. The Spleen and the Kidneys

The relationship between these two zang-organs can be reflected in two aspects: mutual promotion of congenital constitution and acquired constitution, and water metabolism.

1. Mutual Promotion of Congenital Constitution and Acquired Constitution

In the first aspect, on one hand, the spleen transports and transforms food. However, the spleen needs to be aided and promoted by kidney qi, kidney yin and kidney yang. That's why we call that the congenital root warms and nourishes the acquired root. On the other hand, the congenital essence and primordial qi stored in kidney also depend on the supplementation and cultivation of cereal qi and cereal essence which are transformed by spleen qi. That's why we call that the acquired root supplements and cultivates the congenital root.

2. Mutual Promotion of Water Metabolism

In the second aspect, to properly transport and transform water, spleen qi needs the support of kidney, such as the steaming of kidney qi and the warming of kidney yang. Besides, kidney qi controls water metabolism. The work of this function depends on the aid of spleen qi and spleen yang. In a conclusion, the spleen and the kidneys work together to balance water metabolism.

第五节 脏与腑的关系
Section Five The Relationship Between Zang-organs and Fu-organs

脏与腑的关系是通过经脉的相互络属而构成了表里关系。主要有三个方面：①经脉络属；②生理配合；③病理相关。

（1）心与小肠：相互为用。

（2）肺与大肠：主要体现在肺气肃降与大肠传导之间的相互为用关系。

（3）脾与胃：水谷纳运相得，气机升降相因，阴阳燥湿相济。

（4）肝与胆：同司疏泄，共主勇怯。

（5）肾与膀胱：共主小便。

Zang-organs and fu-organs are related internally and externally via meridians. It mainly reflects in three aspects：①they are connected via meridians；②they work together physiologically；③they can influence each other pathologically.

（1）The heart and the small intestines can work together.

（2）The descending function of the lungs and the transmission function of the large intestine can promote and influence each other.

（3）The spleen and the stomach work together to receive and transport food. The ascending function of the spleen and the descending function of the stomach cooperate each other. The spleen likes dampness and the stomach loathes dryness. Therefore，they need to work together.

（4）The liver and the gallbladder work together to soothe and controls courage and timidness.

（5）The kidneys and the bladder control urine together.

第三章　气血津液
Chapter Three　Qi，Blood，Fluids and Liquids

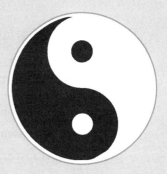

第一节　气
Section One　Qi

一、概念

人体之气，是人体内活力很强、运行不息、无形可见的极精微物质，是构成人体和维持人体生命活动的基本物质之一。

Ⅰ. Definition

The qi in the human body is a vigorous and invisible substance that moves endlessly. It constitutes the human body and maintains life activities.

二、生成

人体之气来源于禀受于父母的先天之精所化生的先天之气，源于饮食物的水谷之精所化生的水谷之气，以及由肺肾吸纳的自然界的清气。

Ⅱ. Generation

Qi is originated from the congenital qi transformed from congenital essence inherited from parents, cereal qi generated from food and drink, and the fresh air inhaled from the nature by the lungs and the kidneys.

三、运动

气的运动称作气机，有升、降、出、入四种形式。由人体之气的运动而引起的精、气、血、津液等物质与能量的新陈代谢过程叫人体气化,是生命最基本的特征之一。

Ⅲ. Movement

Qi moves by ascending, descending, entering and exiting. Along with qi movement, essence, qi, blood and fluids all start metabolism. This metabolism is called qi transformation and it is one of the basic features of life activities.

四、分类

1. 元气

元气是人体最根本、最重要的气,是人体生命活动的原动力。推动和调节人体的生长发育与生殖功能;推动和调控各脏腑、经络、五体、官窍的生理活动。

2. 宗气

宗气是由谷气与自然界清气相结合而积聚于胸中的气,属后天之气的范畴。宗气生成后积聚于胸中,通过上出息道、贯注心脉及沿三焦下行的方式布散全身。

3. 营气

营气是行于脉中而具有营养作用的气,由脾胃运化的水谷之精中精华部分所化生,进入脉中、运行全身。具有化生血液、营养全身的作用。

4. 卫气

卫气是行于脉外而具有保卫作用的气,由脾胃运化的水谷之精中慓悍滑利部分所化生,运行于脉外、布散全身。具有防御外邪、温养全身、调控腠理的作用。

Ⅳ. Classification

1. Primordial Qi

Primordial qi is the most fundamental and most important qi in the human body. As an original driver for life activities, it promotes and regulates growth, development and reproduction. In addition, it also promotes physiological activities of zang-fu organs, meridians and collaterals, five body constituents and orifices.

2. Pectoral Qi

Pectoral qi is the qi that combines cereal qi and fresh air and situates in the chest. After accumulating in the chest, pectoral qi will be distributed all over the body by ascending through respiratory tract, infusing into heart vessels and descending along triple energizers.

3. Nutrient Qi

Nutrient qi is the qi that circulates within vessels and can nourishes the whole body. Stemmed from the smooth part of cereal qi transformed by the spleen and the stomach, nutrient qi enters into the vessels and circulates around the whole body. It can generate blood and nourish the whole body.

4．Defensive Qi

Defensive qi is the qi that flows on the out layer of the body and can defend the whole body. Stemmed from the coarse part of cereal qi transformed by the spleen and the stomach, defensive qi is on the exterior and all over the body. It can ward off pathogens, warm the body and regulate the striae (of skin, muscles and viscera).

第二节　血
Section Two　Blood

一、概念

血是循行于脉中而富有营养的红色液态物质，是构成人体和维持人体生命活动的基本物质之一。

Ⅰ. Definition

Blood is a red fluid that is rich in nutrients and flows in the vessels. It is one of the basic substances to constitute human body and maintain life activities.

二、生成

由水谷之精化生的营气和津液是化生血液的主要物质基础，也是血液的主要构成成分。肾精充足，则可化为肝血以充实血液。此外，肾精化生髓，精髓是化生血液的基本物质之一。

Ⅱ. Generation

Nutrient qi transformed by cereal essence and fluids are the main substances for the generation of blood, and also the main components of blood. If kidney essence is sufficient, the essence can be transformed into liver blood for supplementation. In addition, kidney essence can also be transformed into marrows. Therefore, marrow is also one of the substances.

三、功能

血的主要功能是濡养、化神。

Ⅲ. Functions

The main functions of blood are to nourish and to be transformed into shen.

四、运行

心气的推动、肺气的宣降、肝气的疏泄是推动和促进血液运行的重要因素。脾气的统摄和肝气的藏血是固摄控制血液运行的重要因素。而心、肺、肝、脾等脏生理功能的相互协调与密切配合，共同保证了血液的正常运行。

Ⅳ. Movement

The circulation of blood depends on the propelling of heart qi, diffusing and descending of lung qi and the soothing of liver qi. Meanwhile, spleen qi controls the blood in the vessels and liver qi stores blood, which are the essential factors for controlling the blood circulation. Therefore, the heart, the lungs, the liver and the spleen need to work together and collaborate with each other to ensure the normal circulation of blood.

第三节　津　液
Section Three　Fluids and Liquids

一、概念

津液，是机体一切正常水液的总称（包括各脏腑形体官窍的内在液体及其正常的分泌物，如唾、涎、涕、泪和胃液、肠液、关节腔液、胸腹腔等间隙的液体等），是构成人体和维持人体生命活动的基本物质之一。

Ⅰ. Definition

Fluids and liquids refer to all normal water in the body (including the fluids in zang-fu organs, body constituents and orifices, the normal excreta, such as saliva, spittle, snivel, tear, gastric juice, intestinal juice, and fluids in articular cavity, thorax and abdominal cavity). It is one of the basic substances to constitute the human body and to maintain life activities.

二、功能

津液的主要功能是滋润濡养和充养血脉。另外，津液的代谢对调节机体内外环境的阴阳相对平衡起着十分重要的作用。

Ⅱ. Functions

Fluids and liquids are to moisten and to nourish vessels. In addition, their metabolism also plays an important role in balancing yin and yang of the body.

第四节　气、血、津液之间的关系
Section Four　The Relationship Among Qi，Blood，Fluids and Liquids

一、气与血的关系

1. 气为血之帅

气能生血,血液的化生离不开气作为动力,营气在血液生成中起作用。气能行血,血液的运行离不开气的推动作用。气能摄血,血液能正常循行于脉中,离不开气的固摄作用。

2. 血为气之母

血能养气,气的充盛及其功能发挥离不开血液的濡养。血能载气,气存于血中,依赖血的运载而运行全身。

Ⅰ. The Relationship Between Qi and Blood

1. Qi is the Commander of Blood

Qi can generate blood, for qi, especially the nutrient qi, is a driver for the generation of blood. Qi can promote blood circulation. The blood cannot circulate without the propelling of qi. Qi can control blood. To circulate within the vessels, blood needs the controlling function of qi.

2. Blood is the Mother of Qi

Blood nourishes qi. The nourishment of blood is essential to the exuberance of qi and the full play of qi. Blood carries qi. Qi exists in blood and it circulates along with blood.

二、血与津液的关系

精血同源,津液和血来源相同而又可有相互滋生、相互转化的关系。

Ⅱ. The Relationship Between Blood and Fluids and Liquids

Essence and blood share a common source. Fluids and liquids have a similar source with blood. Besides, they can generate and transform to each other.

第四章 经 络
Chapter Four Meridians and Collaterals

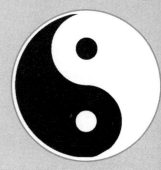

第一节 经络学说概况
Section One The Theory of Meridians and Collaterals

一、基本概念

经络，是经脉和络脉的总称，是运行全身气血、联络脏腑形体官窍、沟通上下内外、感应传导信息的通路系统，是人体结构的重要组成部分。

Ⅰ. Definition

Meridians and collaterals are the channels to carry qi and blood, connect zang-fu organs to body constitutes and orifices, communicate the upper with the lower, the internal with the external, and to response to the transmitting signals. They are important components for the human body.

二、组成

经脉包括正经、经别和奇经。络脉包括别络、孙络和浮络。连属部分：经络在体内连属于脏腑，在体表连属于筋肉、关节和皮肤，包括经筋和皮部。

Ⅱ. Components

Meridians involve twelve regular meridians, meridian divergence and their branches. Collaterals involve divergent collaterals, minute collateral and superficial collaterals. Connecting part: meridians internally connect zang-fu organs and link to muscles, joints and skin at the surface of the body. Therefore, the connecting parts involve meridian sinew and cutaneous regions.

三、经络的生理功能

（1）经络在机体整体统一性的形成中，起到了沟通联系的作用。

（2）运输渗灌气血，使各脏腑、五体、官窍及经络自身得到气血的充分温煦、濡养，而能发挥其各自的功能。

（3）具有感应及传导针灸或其他刺激等各种信息的作用。

（4）经络系统通过其沟通联系、运输渗灌气血作用及其经气对信息的感受、负载和传递作用，能够调节各脏腑五体官窍的功能活动，使人体复杂的生理功能相互协调，维持机体阴阳动态平衡状态。

Ⅲ. Physiological Functions of Meridians and Collaterals

（1）Meridians and colleterals connect the body parts into a whole.

（2）Meridians and collaterals are infused with qi and blood. Therefore, zang-fu organs, five body constituents, orifices and even meridians themselves can be warmed and nourished by qi and blood so that they can work properly.

（3）Meridians and collaterals can response to acupuncture, moxibustion and any other stimuli.

（4）Through the functions mentioned above, meridians and collaterals can regulate the functions of zang-fu organs, five body constituents and orifices, coordinate the complicated functions of each body part and maintain the dynamic equilibrium of the body.

四、经络的应用

阐释病理变化、指导疾病的诊断、指导疾病的治疗。

Ⅳ. Application

Meridians and collaterals can explain the pathological changes and guide the diagnosis and treatment.

第二节　十二经脉
Section Two　Twelve Regular Meridians

一、概念

十二正经即手三阴经（肺、心包、心）、手三阳经（大肠、三焦、小肠）、足三阳经（胃、胆、膀胱）、足三阴经（脾、肝、肾）

Ⅰ. Definition

Twelve regular meridians refer to three hand yin meridians（lung meridian, pericardium meridian, heart meridian）, three hand yang meridians（large intestine meridian, triple energizers and small intestine meridian）, three foot yang meridians（stomach meridian, gallbladder meridian, bladder meridian）, three foot yin meridians（spleen meridian, liver meridian, kidney meridian）.

二、走向

手三阴经从胸走手；手三阳经从手上头；足三阳经从头走足；足三阴经从足至腹胸。

Ⅱ. Running Directions

Three hand yin meridians run from the chest to the hand; three hand yang meridians from the hand to the head; three foot yang meridians from the head to the foot; three foot yin meridians from the foot to the abdomen and the chest.

三、交接规律

表里的阴阳经在四肢末端交接；同名阳经在头面部交接；相互衔接的阴经在胸中交接。

Ⅲ. Connection

Yang meridians link to yin meridians that are internally and externally connected at the extremities of four limbs; yang meridians with the same name are joined together at the head and the face; yin meridians are joined together at the chest.

四、分布规律

左右对称地分布于头面、躯干和四肢。阳经（属六腑）分布于头面、躯干及四肢外侧，阴经(归五脏)分布于胸腹及四肢内侧手经分布于上肢。

Ⅳ. Distribution

Twelve regular meridians are symmetrically distributed at the head and face, trunk and four limbs. Yang meridians (pertaining to six fu-organs) are at the head, face, the lateral side of trunk and four limbs, while yin meridians (pertaining to five zang-organs) are at the chest, abdomen and medial side of four limbs (hand yin meridians are at the upper limbs).

五、表里属络关系

十二经脉在体内与脏腑相属络;阴经属脏主里络腑,阳经属腑主表络脏;一脏配一腑,一阴配一阳,构成脏腑相表里属络关系。

Ⅴ. Connections

Twelve regular meridians are associated with the zang-fu organs in the body. Yin meridians pertain to the internal and are linked to fu-organs, while yang meridians pertain to the external and are linked to zang-organs. One zang-organ is connected to one fu-organ, so one yin meridian is linked internally and externally to one yang meridian.

第三节　奇经八脉
Section Three　Eight Extra Meridians

一、概念

奇经八脉,是指不同于十二正经的八条经脉,即督脉、任脉、冲脉、带脉、阴跷脉、阳跷脉、阴维脉和阳维脉。

Ⅰ. Definition

Eight extra meridians refer to eight improtant meridians that are different from twelve regular meridians. They are governor vessel, conception vessel, thoroughfare vessel, belt vessel, yin heel vessel, yang heel vessel, yin link vessel and yang link vessel.

二、主要生理作用

密切十二经脉的联系,调节十二经脉气血,与某些脏腑关系密切(奇经八脉在循行分布过程中与脑、髓、女子胞等奇恒之腑以及肾脏等有较为密切的联系）。

Ⅱ. Main Physiological Functions

Eight extra meridians closely associate with twelve regular meridians, so they can regulate the qi and blood of regular meridians. In addition, they are closely related with some zang-fu organs. Their running route links kidneys and some extraordinary organs, such as brain, marrow and uterus.

三、督脉

督脉为"阳脉之海"，调节阳经气血；可反映脑、髓和肾的功能。

Ⅲ. Governor Vessel

Governor vessel is called "the sea of yang meridians", so it can regulate qi and blood of yang meridians. It can reflect the functions of brain, marrow and kidneys.

四、任脉

任脉为"阴脉之海"，调节阴经气血；任主胞胎。

Ⅳ. Conception Vessel

Conception vessel is regarded as "the sea of yin meridians", so it can regulate qi and blood of yin meridians. It controls uterus and conception.

五、冲脉

冲脉为"十二经脉之海""五脏六腑之海"，能调节十二经脉及五脏六腑气血；为"血海"，与女子月经及孕育功能有关；与男子的性、生殖功能也有密切的关系。

Ⅴ. Thoroughfare Vessel

Thoroughfare vessel is considered as the sea of twelve regular meridians and the sea of five zang-organs and six fu-organs. Therefore, it can regulate the qi and blood of these meridians and organs. In addition, thoroughfare vessel is also called the sea of blood and it is related to the menstruation, conception, and the sex and the reproduction of the male.

六、带脉

常脉约束纵行诸经；主司妇女带下；维络腰腹，提系胞胎和固护胎儿。

VI. Belt Vessel

Belt vessel constrains meridians that run longitudinally. It controls vaginal discharge, supports waist, abdomen and uterus, and protects fetus.

七、阴、阳跷脉

阴、阳跷脉主司下肢运动;司眼睑开合。

VII. Yin Heel Vessel and Yang Heel Vessel

Yin heel vessel and yang heel vessel control the movement of lower limbs and the opening and closing of eyelids.

八、阴、阳维脉

阳维脉具有维系、联络全身阳经的作用,阴维脉具有维系、联络全身阴经的作用。在正常情况下,阴、阳维脉互相维系,对气血盛衰起调节溢蓄作用,而不参与环流。

VIII. Yin Link Vessel and Yang Link Vessel

Yang link vessel supports and links all yang meridians, while yin link vessel supports and links all yin meridians. Under the normal conditions, both vessels support each other and regulate qi and blood. But they are not involved in the circulation.

第四节   其他组成部分
Section Four   Other Components

一、经别

经别是十二正经别行深入体腔的支脉。

I. Meridian Divergence

Meridian divergence refers to the branches of twelve regular meridians that run deeply in the body.

二、别络

十二经脉和任、督二脉各自别出一络,加上脾之大络,总计 15 条称为十五络脉(别络)。

Ⅱ. Divergent Collaterals

Twelve regular meridians, conception vessel and governor vessel all have one divergent collateral, respectively. In addition to the great collateral of the spleen, there are fifteen divergent collaterals all together.

三、经筋

经筋是指十二经脉之气濡养筋肉、骨节的体系，是附属于十二经脉的筋膜系统。

Ⅲ. Meridians Sinew

Meridians sinew is a system of muscles, tendons, sinews, bones and joints nourished by the qi of twelve regular meridians. It affiliates to the sinew membranes of regular meridians.

四、皮部

十二皮部是十二经脉功能活动反映于体表的部位，也是络脉之气散布之所在。

Ⅳ. Cutaneous Regions

Twelve cutaneous regions refer to the regions in the surface of body that reflect the functions of twelve regular meridians. They are the place where the qi of collaterals is distributed.

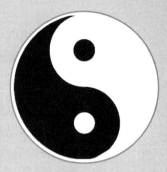

第五章 病因病机
Chapter Five　Etiology and Pathogenesis

第一节　病　因
Section One　Etiology

一、外感病因

外感病因主要包括六淫和疠气两个方面。

1. 六淫

在正常情况下,风、寒、暑、湿、燥、火是自然界的六种气候变化,称为"六气"。六气的正常运行变化,有利于万物的生长变化,但如果六气太过或不及,则气候反常。在人体抵抗力低下时,就能成为致病因素,则称"六淫"或"六邪"。

2. 疠气

疠气,是一类具有强烈致病性和传染性的外感病邪。致病特点:①发病急骤,病情危笃;②传染性强,易于流行;③一气一病,症状相似。

Ⅰ. External Pathogenic Factors

External pathogenic factors mainly involve six climatic pathogens and pestilence.

1. Six Climatic Pathogens

Wind, cold, summer heat, dampness, dryness and fire are six normal climatic factors in the nature. The normal changes of these six factors are beneficial to the growth of beings. If these factors are excessive or deficient, the climate will change. Or when the body resistance is too weak to adapt to the climatic changes, these factors also become pathogens. In this case, six normal climatic changes are called six climatic pathogens or six evils.

2. Epidemic Pathogen

Epidemic pathogen is a kind of fulminating infectious pathogenic factors. Diseases caused by pestilence are often highly infectious with a sudden onset. Although one pestilence factor will cause one kind of disease, the symptoms are similar.

二、内伤病因

七情内伤，是指喜、怒、忧、思、悲、恐、惊七种引发或诱发疾病的情志活动。致病特点：①直接伤及内脏；②影响脏腑气机，气机失调又可妨碍机体的气化过程，引起精气血津液的代谢失常，从而继发多种病证。

II. Internal Pathogenic Factors

Internal damages caused by seven emotions refer to diseases resulted from or triggered by joy, anger, anxiety, contemplation, grief, fear and fright. These emotional factors attack internal organs directly and affect qi movements. Disordered qi movements also affect qi transformation, causing the abnormal metabolism of essence, qi, blood, fluids and liquids and further leading to diseases.

三、病理产物形成的病因

是指在疾病过程中由于脏腑精气血津液功能失调所形成的病理产物，又成为新的病证发生的病因。病理产物形成的病因可分为痰饮、瘀血和结石三大类。

1. 痰饮

痰饮是人体水液输布、排泄障碍所形成的又能导致多种病证的病理产物。外感六淫，或七情内伤，或饮食不宜，或劳逸失度等，使肺、脾、肾、肝及三焦等脏腑气化功能失常，以致水液输布、排泄障碍、水液停聚而形成。致病特点：阻滞气血运行，影响水液代谢，易于蒙蔽清窍、扰乱心神，致病广泛、变幻多端。

2. 瘀血

瘀血是指丧失了正常功能、不为生理上所需要的瘀积之血，包括体内瘀积的离经之血，以及因血行不畅而停滞于脉内之血。瘀血既是疾病过程中所形成的病理产物，又是某些疾病的致病因素。成因：血出、气滞、虚、血寒、血热都会致瘀。此外，还有"久病从瘀"之说。致病的病证特点：疼痛、肿块、出血、色紫黯，可表现出肌肤甲错及脉象上的某些异常，如涩脉或结代脉等。

III. Pathological Substances

Pathological substances are caused by dysfunctions of zang-fu organs, essence, qi, blood, fluids and liquids. However, these substances, such as phlegm-retained fluid, blood stasis and lithiasis, can also be the causes of diseases.

1. Phlegm-retained Fluid

Phlegm-retained fluid is the pathological substances caused by disorders in water metabolism and distribution. Due to six evils, seven emotion, improper diet, overstrain or the dysfunction of qi transformation of the lungs, the spleen, the kidneys, the liver and triple energizers, the distribution of body fluids is influenced and fluids are retained. The diseases resulting from them are often changeable, obstructing the circulation of qi and blood, influencing water metabolism, clouding the clear orifices and even disturbing the mind.

2. Blood Stasis

Blood stasis refers to the blood without the normal functions and unnecessary for physiological needs. It contains the extravasated blood which is accumulated in the body and retained blood due to stagnated circulation. Blood stasis can be a pathological substance that can lead to other diseases. Bleeding, qi stagnation, qi deficiency, blood cold and blood heat can all lead to stasis. Long-term diseases can also result in stasis. Blood stasis frequently causes pain, swellings, bleeding, cyanosis, squamous and dry skin and abnormal pulses, such as unsmooth pulse and knotted and intermittent pulse.

第二节 病 机
Section Two Pathogenesis

病机,即疾病发生、发展与变化的机制。

Pathogenesis refers to the mechanism involved in the onset, development and changes of diseases.

一、邪正盛衰

邪正盛衰,是指在疾病过程中,邪正之间相互斗争,双方在力量对比上所发生的消长盛衰变化。

Ⅰ. The Struggle Between Evils and Body Resistance

During the course of a disease, evils and body resistances will fight against each other. In such a combat, superabundance or decline between body resistance and evils leads to diseases.

二、阴阳失调

阴阳失调即阴阳之间失去平衡协调的简称,是指在疾病的发生、发展过程中,由于各种致病因素的影响,导致机体的阴阳双方失去相对的平衡协调而出现的阴阳偏胜、偏衰、互损、格拒、亡失等一系列病理变化。

II. Disharmony Between Yin and Yang

Disharmony between yin and yang refers to the fact that during the occurrence and development of diseases, various causes will unbalance yin and yang, leading to predominance, decline, mutual consumption, repulsion or even depletion of yin and yang.

三、气、血、津液失常

气的失常包括气虚、气滞、气逆、气陷、气闭和气脱。血的失常包括血虚、血瘀、出血、血寒和血热。津液代谢失常包括津液不足、津液输布、排泄障碍和津液与气血关系失调。

III. Abnormalities of Qi, Blood, Fluids and Liquids

Abnormalities of qi involve qi deficiency, qi stagnation, qi reversal, qi sinking, qi blockage and qi collapse. Abnormalities of blood contain blood deficiency, blood stasis, bleeding, blood cold and blood heat. Abnormalities of fluids and liquids consist of insufficiency, distribution disorders, discharge problems, disharmony between body fluids and qi, and imbalance between body fluids and blood.

四、内生"五邪"

内生"五邪"(又称内生"五气"),是指在疾病的发展过程中,由于脏腑经络及精气血津液的功能失常所产生的,在临床表现上与风、寒、湿、燥、火等六淫外邪致病相类似的五种病理变化;包括内风、内寒、内湿、内燥和内火(内热)等。

IV. Five Internal Evils

Five internal evils, also called five internal qi, refer to five pathological changes caused by dysfunction of zang-fu organs, meridians and collaterals, qi, blood and body fluids. These changes are like those caused by six evils, such as wind, cold, dampness, dryness and fire. Therefore, these internal changes are called internal wind, internal cold, internal dampness, internal dryness and internal fire (internal heat).

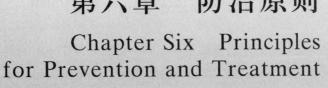

第六章　防治原则
Chapter Six　Principles for Prevention and Treatment

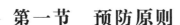

第一节　预防原则
Section One　Principles for Prevention

一、未病先防

未病先防是指在未病之前,采取各种措施,做好预防工作,以防止疾病的发生。措施是养生以增强正气,防止病邪侵害。

Ⅰ. Prevention Before Onset of Disease

Prevention before onset of diseases means that before the occurrence, measures, such as strengthening of body resistance and prevention of evil attack, should be taken to prevent the onset of diseases.

二、既病防变

既病防变,是指在疾病发生的初始阶段,应力求做到早期诊断、早期治疗,以防止疾病的发展及传变。措施是早期诊治,防止传变。

Ⅱ. To Prevent Exacerbation After Being Ill

To prevent exacerbation after being ill means that at the initial stage of disease, early diagnosis and timely treatment should be guaranteed to prevent the progress and exacerbation of diseases.

第二节　治疗原则
Section Two　Principles for Treatment

治则是指治疗疾病时所必须遵循的基本原则。治法是指在一定治则指导下制订的针对疾病与症候的具体治疗大法、治疗方法及治疗措施。包括正治与反治、治标与治本、扶正与祛邪、调整阴阳、调理精气血津液和三因制宜等。

Therapeutic principle refers to the basic principles that need to be conformed to during the treatment of diseases. Therapeutic methods refer to therapeutic approaches and measures specifically for a disease or a pattern under the guidance of therapeutic principles. Therapeutic principles involve routine treatment and contrary treatment, treating superficial symptoms and treating the root, strengthening the body resistance and expelling evils, balancing yin and yang, regulating essence, qi, blood and body fluids, treatment in accordance with triple etiologies (season, locality and individual).

一、正治

正治是指采用与疾病的证候性质相反的方药以治疗的一种治疗原则。主要内容包括寒者热之、热者寒之、虚则补之、实则泻之。

Ⅰ. Routine Treatment

Routine treatment for opposite symptoms refers to the therapeutic principle for treating diseases with drugs that have the opposite nature with the disease nature. It involves treating cold syndrome with hot-natured drugs, treating heat syndrome with cold-natured drugs, treating deficiency syndrome with supplementing method, and purging in excess case.

二、反治

反治是指顺从病证的外在假象而治的一种治疗原则。主要内容包括热因热用、寒因寒用、塞因塞用、通因通用。

Ⅱ. Contrary Treatment

Contrary treatment refers to the therapeutic principle for treating a disease with drugs coinciding with the pseudo-symptom. It contains treating false-heat syndrome with hot-natured drugs, treating false-cold syndrome with cold-natured drugs, treating obstructive syndrome with nourishing therapy, treating diarrhea with purgatives.

三、治标与治本

缓则治本：即指在病情缓和,病势迁延,暂无急重病状的情况下,必须着眼于疾病本质的治疗。急则治标：指标病急重,应当先治、急治其标病。标本兼治：即指标本并重或标本均不太急时,应当标本同时治疗。

Ⅲ. Treating Superficial Symptoms and Treating the Root

When the disease is mild and chronic and it is unlikely to worsen at the moment, the treatment should focus on the disease root. When the disease is acute, the focus should be on the symptoms. When the symptoms and root are not acute, both the symptom and the root need to be treated simultaneously.

四、扶正祛邪

扶正是指扶助正气、增强体质、提高机体的抗邪及康复能力的一种治疗原则。祛邪是指祛除邪气、消解病邪的侵袭和损害、抑制亢奋有余的病理反应的一种治疗原则。

Ⅳ. Strengthening Body Resistance and Expelling Evils

Strengthening body resistance refers to a therapeutic principle to support healthy qi, strengthen body constitution, increase the ability to ward off diseases and to rehabilitate; expelling evils refers to the principle to eliminate pathogenic factors.

五、调整阴阳

损其有余适用于人体阴或阳偏盛所致的实寒证或实热证的治则。补其不足适用于人体阴阳偏衰或阴阳互损所致病证的治则。

Ⅴ. Balancing Yin and Yang

To purge the excess is a therapeutic principle for excess-cold pattern or excess-heat pattern caused by predominance of yin or yang. To supplement the insufficiency is a therapeutic principle for yin deficiency, yang deficiency or mutual consumption of yin and yang.

六、调理精气血津液

Ⅵ. Regulating Essence, Qi, Blood and Body Fluids

根据气与血、气与津液、气与精以及精血津液之间的病理关系,进行相应的调整。

Relevant regulation should be given according to the pathological relationships between qi and blood, qi and body fluids, qi and essence, essence and blood, and blood and body fluids.

七、三因制宜

因时制宜是指根据时令气候节律特点，来制订适宜的治疗原则。因时之"时"，一指自然界的时令气候特点，二指年、月、日的时间变化规律。因地制宜是指根据不同的地域环境特点，来制订适宜的治疗原则。因人制宜是指根据病人的年龄、性别、体质等不同特点，来制订适宜的治疗原则。

Ⅶ. Treatment in Accordance with Triple Etiologies

Treatment in accordance with seasonal conditions refers to the principle to treat according to the climate characteristics of different seasons, or the changes of year, month and day. Treatment in accordance with local conditions means to treat on the basis of features of different locations. Treatment in accordance with the patient's individuality refers to the principle to treat based on patient's age, gender, body constitution and other individual features.

第二部分
推 拿
Part Two Tuina

推拿手法,是指以治疗或保健为目的,用手或肢体其他部分刺激受术部位或活动肢体的规范化的技巧动作。推拿手法要求持久、有力、均匀、柔和,从而达到深透。"持久",是指手法能按照规定的技术要求和操作规范持续运用一段时间,保持动作和力量的连贯性,不变形走样,不断断续续;"有力",是指手法必须具有一定的力量,这种力量不是固定不变的,而应该根据病人体质、病证虚实、治疗部位和手法性质等不同情况而增减;"均匀",是指手法动作的节奏性和用力的平稳性。手法的动作频率、压力或幅度都应该保持相对一致,频率不要时快时慢,压力不要时轻时重,幅度不要忽大忽小;"柔和"是指手法操作平稳缓和、轻重得宜和动作变换的自然协调,使手法轻而不浮,重而不滞。以上各点是有机联系的。

　　Tuina manipulations are standardized techniques including the use of hand or other parts of limbs to work on the lesion or to move limbs with the purpose of treatment or health care. The requirements of tuina manipulation are being lasting, powerful, uniform and gentle. Being lasting refers to that the manipulation works as required for some time with stable movement and constant strength. Being powerful refers to doing tuina with strength which adapts to the patient's physique, the characters of diseases, the site of focus and the manipulations, instead of keeping the strength constant. Being uniform refers to the rhythm of manipulation and the stability of strength. The frequency, strength, and range of manipulations should be the same relatively all the time. Being gentle refers to keeping the manipulations comfortable, which requires appropriate frequency, strength and range as well as coordination while the manipulation is changed. All the requirements above are connected with each other.

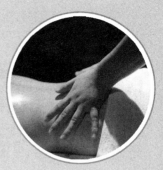

第七章 推拿常用手法
Chapter Seven Commonly-used Tuina Manipulations

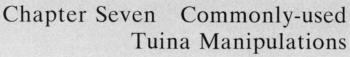

第一节 一指禅推法
Section One Qi-concentrated Single-finger Pushing Manipulation

一、概念

用拇指指端、指纹面或偏锋着力于受术部位或穴位上，以肘部为支点，前臂作主动摆动，带动腕部摆动和拇指关节做屈伸活动，称为"一指禅推法"。

Ⅰ. Definition

Operator uses the tip or the side of the thumb, or the whorled surface of the thumb to push the region to be treated. Forearm sways with elbow as the fulcrum, with combined movement of the wrist swaying and thumb flexion and extension. It is so called "qi-concentrated single-finger pushing manipulation".

二、动作要领

用拇指指端、指纹面或偏锋着力于受术部位或穴位上，沉肩、垂肘、悬腕、掌虚、指实，前臂作主动摆动，带动腕部摆动和拇指关节作屈伸活动。手法频率为每分钟 120—160 次。

Ⅱ. Requirements

The operator uses the tip or the side of the thumb, or the whorled surface of the thumb to push the region to be treated, with the shoulders lowered, the elbow dropped, the wrist lifted, the palm relaxed and the thumb tensed. The forearm sways with the elbow as the fulcrum, with combined movements of the wrist swaying and the thumb flexion and extension. The frequency is 120 – 160 times/min.

三、注意事项

摆动时,尺侧要低于桡侧;压力、频率、摆动幅度要均匀,动作要灵活;坐位练习和操作时,肘关节略低于手腕;临床应用时应注意拇指自然着力,不可用蛮力下压。一指禅推法的频率加快到每分钟 200 次以上称为缠法。

Ⅲ. Notes

The pressure, the frequency, and the range of swing should keep regular with flexible action. You should flexibly manipulate with balanced tension, frequency and range. When you practice and operate in sitting position, you should put the elbow joint lower than the wrist. Clinically, you should press the thumb naturally without pressing in a brute force. The frequency at more than 200 times/min is called quick pushing manipulation (Chan Fa).

四、临床应用

本法具有舒筋活络,调和营卫,行气活血,健脾和胃等作用。适用于全身各部和穴位。临床上常用于治疗头痛、失眠、面瘫、胃痛、腹痛及关节筋骨酸痛等病证。

Ⅳ. Clinical Application

The manipulation can stimulate the circulation of the blood and relax the muscles and joints, harmonize nutrient qi and defensive qi, promote qi to activate blood, and strengthen the spleen and stomach. It can be used on the whole body and every acupoint. Clinically, it is usually used for headache, insomnia, facial paralysis, stomachache, abdominal pain, and joints and muscles ache.

第二节　揉　法
Section Two　Rolling Manipulation

一、概念

揉法由丁季峰所创。揉法是由腕关节的伸屈运动和前臂的旋转运动复合而成。

Ⅰ. Definition

Created by Ding Jifeng, rolling manipulation is made up of wrist extension and flexion and forearm rotation.

二、动作要领

以小指掌指关节背侧点附着于受术部位,以肘部为支点,前臂作主动摆动,带动腕部伸屈和前臂旋转的复合运动,使手掌背侧近小指部分在受术部位上持续不断地来回滚动。手法频率为每分钟 140 次左右。

Ⅱ. Requirements

Put the dorsal side of the little finger joint on the operated place. With the elbow as the fulcrum, actively swing the forearm to drive the composite movements of wrist extension and flexion and the forearm rotation, making the dorsal side of the palm continue to roll back and forth on the operated place. The frequency of the manipulation is about 140 times/min.

三、注意事项

本法的特点是滚动摩擦,滚动时掌背尺侧要紧贴体表,不能拖动、辗转或跳动。压力、频率和摆动幅度要均匀,动作要协调而有节律。肩臂不要过分紧张,肘关节屈曲 100°—120°,肘部离开身体约 15 cm。各手指任其自然,不宜过度屈曲或伸直;要压力平稳、动作协调、节奏均匀。

Ⅲ. Notes

The manipulation is characterized by rolling friction. When to operate rolling manipulation, you should put the ulnar side of palm back close to the body surface, without dragging, tossing or beating. Pressure, frequency and amplitude of swinging should be uniform, and the action should be coordinated and rhythmic. The shoulder and arm should not be too rigid. Flexion of the elbow should be within 100 degrees to 120 degrees and the elbow should be about 15cm away from the body. Each finger should be at nature status without excessive flexion or extension. The pressure should be steady; the movement should be coordinated and the rhythm should be even.

四、临床应用

本法具有舒筋活血、滑利关节等作用,适用于肩背腰臀及四肢等肌肉较丰厚的部位。对风湿酸痛、麻木不仁、肢体瘫痪、运动功能障碍等疾患常用本法治疗。

Ⅳ. Clinical Application

The manipulation can stimulate the circulation of the blood, relax the muscles and joints, lubricate joint and so on. It can be used for shoulders, back, waist, buttocks and limbs where the muscle is very strong. It can treat rheumatic pain, numbness, paralysis of limbs, motor dysfunction and other diseases.

第三节 揉 法
Section Three Kneading Manipulation

一、概念

分掌揉和指揉两种。掌揉法包括鱼际揉和掌根揉。指揉法有一指揉、二指揉等。鱼际揉法可以摆动操作,也可以旋转操作。

Ⅰ. Definition

It is divided into palm kneading and finger kneading. Palm kneading includes thenar kneading and palm root kneading. Finger kneading includes one finger kneading and two finger kneading, etc. Thenar eminence kneading can be either swinging or rotating.

二、动作要领

摆动式的鱼际揉法要求以鱼际部吸定于受术部位上,腕部放松,以肘部为支点,前臂作主动摆动,带动腕部作轻柔缓和的揉动。其他非摆动式的揉法是以鱼际、掌根或手法指纹面吸定于受术者部位或穴位,带动皮下组织作轻柔缓和的环旋运动。

Ⅱ. Requirements

Thenar eminence kneading of swinging type should put thenar eminence to operated place. You should relax the wrist and swing forearm actively to drive the wrist to knead gently with elbow as a fulcrum. Other non-swinging kneading manipulations would put thenar eminence, palm root or fingerprint side on operated place to drive the subcutaneous tissue to rotate gently.

三、注意事项

摆动式的鱼际揉法归入摆动类手法。揉法必须吸定表皮,带动皮下组织,不可在表皮摩擦。摆动式鱼际揉法的频率为每分钟 120—160 次。揉法操作时压力要轻柔,动作要协调而有节律。

Ⅲ. Notes

Thenar eminence kneading of swinging type belongs to swinging manipulation. Kneading manipulation must be fixed on the skin to drive subcutaneous tissue without friction on the skin. The frequency of this manipulation should be 120 to 160 times/min. When operating kneading manipulation, the pressure should be soft and the action should be coordinated and rhythmic.

四、临床应用

本法具有宽胸理气、活血化瘀、消积导滞、消肿止痛之功,适用于全身各部。常用于脘腹痛、胸胁闷痛、便秘、泄泻等肠胃疾病,以及因外伤引起的红肿疼痛等症。

Ⅳ. Clinical Application

This manipulation can relieve depression in the chest, regulate the flow of qi, activate blood circulation to dissipate blood stasis, eliminate stagnation and relieve swelling and pain. It can be used throughout the body. It is usually used for abdominal pain, chest stuffy pain, constipation, diarrhea, other gastrointestinal diseases and other swollen pain caused by trauma.

第四节　摩　法
Section Four　Rubbing Manipulation

一、概念

以手掌或手指在受术部位作环旋而有节律的抚摩的手法称为摩法。分掌摩和指摩两种。指摩法有单指摩和三指摩等。

Ⅰ. Definition

Using your palm or finger to do annular and rhythmic stroke on operation part is called rubbing manipulation. It is divided into two kinds: palm rubbing and finger rubbing. Finger rubbing includes one-finger rubbing and three-finger rubbing, etc.

二、动作要领

掌摩法是指用掌面附着于受术者部位上,腕关节放松,作环形而有节律性的环旋运动；指摩是手指指纹面附着于受术部位或穴位上，以腕关节为中心，连同掌指作节律性的环旋运动。频率每分钟120次左右。

Ⅱ. Requirements

Palm rubbing manipulation is a kind of annular and rhythmic circumduction which orders your palm to stick to the operation part and your wrist relax. Finger rubbing manipulation needs your fingerprints stick to the body position or acupoints. Then focus on your wrist and do rhythmic circumduction with your finger and palm. The frequency is about 120 times/min.

三、注意事项

摩法操作时肘关节自然屈曲，腕部放松。要缓急适中、轻重得宜。正如《石室秘录》所云："摩法不宜急，不宜缓，不宜轻，不宜重，以中和之义施之"。可顺时针和逆时针双向操作。摩法如配合药膏，称为膏摩。

Ⅲ. Notes

When you apply this manipulation, you should curve your elbow naturally and relax your wrist. Rubbing manipulation requires suitable frequency and strength. *Shishi Mi Lu*: "Rubbing manipulation cannot be too quick or too slow, while it also cannot be too weak or too forceful. Appropriate frequency and strength is preferred." Rubbing manipulation is available both clockwise and anticlockwise. Rubbing with unguent is called ointment rubbing.

四、临床应用

本法具有和中理气，消积导滞、调节胃肠蠕动、活血化瘀等作用，是胸腹胁肋部常用手法。多用于脘腹疼痛、气滞及胸胁胀满、消化不良、外伤肿痛等症的治疗。

Ⅳ. Clinical Application

This manipulation can protect the stomach, accelerate digestion, regulate intestinal activity and promote blood circulation to remove blood stasis. It is usually operated on the chest and abdomen to treat abdominal pain, chest inflation, dyspepsia and trauma.

第五节　推　法
Section Five　Pushing Manipulation

一、概念

推法是用手在受术部位作单方向的直线推动,主要有指推法、掌推法、肘推法三种。

Ⅰ. Definition

Using your hand to do straight pushing movement on the operation part is called pushing manipulation. It mainly includes finger pushing manipulation, palm pushing manipulation and elbow pushing manipulation.

二、动作要领

用指、掌或肘着力于受术部位上作单方向的直线推动。

Ⅱ. Requirements

Use your fingers, palm or elbow to do straight pushing movement on the operation part.

三、注意事项

(1) 操作时指掌或肘要紧贴体表,用力要稳,速度要缓慢而均匀。

(2) 指推法可分为指腹推法(拇指指纹面着力)、指侧推法(拇指桡侧着力)、二指推法(食中二指指纹面着力)、分推法(双手拇指指纹面)等。

(3) 掌推法有全掌推法、小鱼际推法、掌根推法等。

(4) 肘推法是以尺骨鹰嘴部着力,在推拿中刺激最强,一般用于感觉迟钝的患者,不要轻易使用。

Ⅲ. Notes

(1) When you operate, your finger, palm or elbow needs to stick to the body surface. Express your force stably and the frequency should be slow and even.

(2) Finger pushing manipulation includes finger-pulp pushing manipulation (thumb fingerprints side stick to the body), finger-side pushing manipulation (radial side of the thumb stick to the body), two-fingers pushing manipulation (index fingerprints and middle fingerprints stick to the body), and forked pushing

manipulation（both two thumb fingerprints stick to the body）.

（3）Palm pushing manipulation includes full-palm pushing manipulation, hypothenar eminence pushing manipulation and heel of hand pushing manipulation.

（4）Elbow pushing manipulation is using the olecranon to stick to the operation part. It is the most stimulating manipulation especially for those who are insensitive and it is not usually performed.

四、临床应用

适用于人体各部位，能提高肌肉的兴奋性，促进血液循环，并有舒筋活络之功。指推法和掌推法适用于肩背、腰臀及四肢部，用于治疗风湿痹痛、筋肉拘急等软组织疾患。肘推法多用于脊柱两侧膀胱经及臀部，治疗顽固性腰腿痛和麻木不仁的风湿痹痛。指侧推法和二指推法多用于小儿推拿。分推法多用于前额、肩胛上部、腹部、掌心等处，治疗内科杂病。

Ⅳ. Clinical Application

It is widely performed on every part of the body. It can improve muscle excitability, promote blood circulation and activate veins. Finger pushing manipulation and palm pushing manipulation are performed on shoulder, back, waist, buttocks and all four limbs. It is used to cure rheumatic arthralgia, cramps and some other soft tissue diseases. Elbow pushing manipulation is performed on both sides of the spine where the bladder meridian locates and buttocks to cure chronic waist-leg pains and rheumatic arthralgia. Finger-side pushing manipulation and two-fingers pushing manipulation are mostly performed in infantile massage. Forked pushing manipulation is usually performed on forehead, regio suprascapularis, abdomen and palm to cure various diseases of internal medicine.

第六节　擦　法
Section Six　Scraping（Embrocation）Manipulation

一、概念

用手掌作直线来回摩擦，称为擦法。主要有以下三种擦法：以全掌接触的称为掌擦法；以鱼际接触的称为鱼际擦法；以小鱼际着力摩擦的小鱼际擦法。

Ⅰ. Definition

Rubbing in a straight line back and forth with palm named scrapping on embrocation. There are mainly three kinds: touching with full palm is called palm-scrubbing manipulation; touching with thenar eminence is called thenar eminence-scrubbing manipulation; touching with hypothenar eminence is called hypothenar eminence-scrubbing manipulation.

二、动作要领

用手掌的全掌、鱼际或小鱼际着力于受术部位,作直线往返摩擦。操作时腕关节伸直,使前臂与手掌接近相平。着力部位要贴于受术体表,以肩关节为支点,上臂主动发力,带动手掌作直线往返运动。频率为每分钟 100—120 次。

Ⅱ. Requirements

Force on the operation position with the full palm, thenar eminence or hypothenar eminence and rub in a straight line back and forth. Straighten the wrist and make the forearm and the palm of your hand at the same level during the operation. Stick to the surface of the body while operation. Make the elbow joint as the fulcrum and push up actively by the upper arm, drive the palm to move in a straight line back and forth. Operate at frequencies between about 100 and 120 times per minute.

三、注意事项

擦法的垂直压力不宜太大,但推动的幅度要大、路线要长。必须直线往返,不可歪斜。要紧贴受术体表移动,用力宜平稳,动作要均匀连续、不可跳动。术者自然呼吸,不可屏气。如直接在裸露的体表摩擦,必须涂适量润滑油或膏摩制剂,既可防止擦破皮肤,又可通过药物的渗透以加强手法的疗效。擦法作用过的局部体表,一般不要再使用其他手法,否则容易造成破皮。

Ⅲ. Notes

The vertical pressure of embrocation manipulation should not be too much, but the range of pushing must be wide and the route must be long. Rub in a straight line back and forth, which cannot be deflected. Press on the operation surface of body and move with stable force. The actions should be uniformly continuous and do not bounce. The manipulator breathes naturally and cannot hold breath. If rubbing directly on naked surface of body, smear enough lubricating oil or mastic to prevent excoriating and to strengthen the effect by permeating the medicine. The surface which has been rubbed should not be operated by other manipulations as it is easy to break the skin.

四、临床应用

本法具有温经通络、活血祛瘀、消肿止痛、健脾和胃等作用。掌擦法多用于上胸部、胁肋部、腰骶部和腹部等；鱼际擦法多用于上肢；侧擦法多用于脊柱两侧、肩背部和腰骶部。本法常用于治疗脏腑虚损及气血功能失常等虚症和寒症，以及四肢伤筋肿痛、气滞血瘀。

Ⅳ. Clinical Application

The manipulation can warm the meridians, unblock the collaterals, activate blood, remove stasis, relieve swelling and pain, and strengthen the spleen and the stomach. Palm-scrubbing manipulation is usually used on the chest, ribs, lumbosacral portion and abdomen, etc. Thenar eminence-scrubbing manipulation is usually used on the upper limb. Latero-scrubbing manipulation is usually used on both sides of the spine, shoulders, back and lumbosacral portion. It is usually used to cure zang-fu deficiency syndrome and cold syndrome caused by qi-blood functional disorder. It can also cure pain of limbs, qi stagnation and blood stasis.

第七节　搓　法
Section Seven　Foulage Manipulation

一、概念

用双手夹住受术部位，相对用力搓揉的方法，称为搓法。

Ⅰ. Definition

Clamping the operation position with two hands with relative twisting and rubbing is called foulage manipulation.

二、动作要领

用双手掌面对称用力夹住受术部位，作方向相反的来回快速搓揉。

Ⅱ. Requirements

Clamp the operation position symmetrically with two palms; twist and rub fast relatively.

三、注意事项

搓动时可同时沿肢体纵轴作上下往返移动,搓动要快,移动要慢。

Ⅲ. Notes

Move up and down along the limb when twisting. Twist fast and move slowly.

四、临床应用

本法适用于四肢和腰背、胁部,以上肢最为常用。搓法是一种辅助手法,一般在上述部位治疗结束时使用,有舒筋解痉、调和气血等作用。

Ⅳ. Clinical Application

The manipulation is used at limbs, lumbar, back and ribs, mostly at upper limbs. As a supplementary manipulations, foulage manipulation is mainly used as an ending technique for treating the position mentioned above. It can relax tendons, resolve spasm and regulate qi and blood.

第八节　抹　法
Section Eight　Thumb-rubbing Manipulation

一、概念

用拇指指纹面在受术体表作曲线移动,称为抹法。

Ⅰ. Definition

Moving curvedly on the operation surface with the fingerprint of thumb is called thumb-rubbing manipulation.

二、动作要领

除拇指外的其余手指固定相应部位,以单手或双手拇指指纹面着力于受术体表,作上下或左右的曲线往返移动。

Ⅱ. Requirements

Fix the fingers on corresponding part except for the thumb. Put one thumb or two thumbs fingerprint on the operation position and move curvedly up and down or left and right.

三、注意事项

抹法的运行路线比较自由,可以单向运动,也可任意往返;可以走弧线,也可作转折,应根据治疗的需要和不同受术部位而灵活运用。抹法可单手操作,也可双手同时操作。用力要平稳缓和,轻而不浮,重而不滞。

Ⅲ. Notes

The moving route of thumb-rubbing manipulation is free. You can move one-way or back and forth at will. You can also move curvedly or turn based on the need of treatment and different operation position. You can operate with one hand or two hands at the same time. Force smoothly, easily, gently but don't be floated, and hard but not retardant.

四、临床应用

本法具有开窍醒神、镇静明目之功。常用于头面、颈项和手掌。可作为头晕头痛、颈项强痛、指掌麻木等症的辅助治疗。

Ⅳ. Clinical Application

It can induce resuscitation, calm and improve eyesight. It is usually used on head, face, neck and palm. It can be used as a supplementary manipulation of dizziness and headache, neck pain and numbness of finger and palm, etc.

第九节　按　法
Section Nine　Pressing Manipulation

一、概念

分为指按法和掌按法两种。手指按压体表,称指按法。手掌按压体表,称掌按法。

Ⅰ. Definition

It is divided into finger-pressing manipulation and palm-pressing manipulation. Using fingers to press the body surface is finger-pressing manipulation. Using palms to press the body surface is palm-pressing manipulation.

二、动作要领

用指端或指腹按压体表,称指按法。用单掌或双掌重叠按压体表,称掌按法。

Ⅱ. Requirements

Using the fingertip or finger pulp to press the body surface is finger-pressing manipulation. Using one palm or two palms overlapped to press the body is palm-pressing manipulation.

三、注意事项

操作时着力部位要紧贴体表,不可移动;用力要由轻到重,再由重到轻,不可突然加压或减压;指按和掌按操作时往往要借用上身的力量;操作时往往与揉法结合,组成"按揉"复合手法。

Ⅲ. Notes

The point forced should cling to the body surface when manipulating. It can't be moved. The force should be from small to large, then from large to small. We can't add the pressure or reduce the pressure suddenly. Usually, we rely on the weight of our upper body when using finger-pressing and palm-pressing manipulation. We usually combine it with kneading manipulation, forming them into compound manipulation.

四、临床应用

本法具有放松肌肉、活血止痛之功。指按法适用于全身各部穴位,掌按法多用于腰背部、腹部、股后部等。常用于治疗胃脘痛、头痛、肢体酸痛麻木等病证。

Ⅳ. Clinical Application

Clinically, using this manipulation has functions to relax muscles, activate blood and alleviate pain. Finger-pressing manipulation is applicable to all acupuncture points on the whole body, and palm-pressing manipulation is usually applied on the lower back, the abdomen and the back of buttock, etc. It is commonly used to treat epigastralgia, headache, numbness of the limbs and ache, etc.

第十节　点　法
Section Ten　Pointing Manipulation

一、概念

用指端或屈曲的指间关节垂直按压受术部位的手法，称为点法。点法分为拇指点法和屈指点法两种。

Ⅰ．Definition

The manipulation refers to vertical pressing of the therapeutic region with fingertip or inflectional interphalangeal joints. It can be divided into thumb pointing manipulation and inflectional-finger pointing manipulation.

二、动作要领

拇指点法是用拇指指端按压受术体表；屈指点法是用屈曲的拇指指间关节桡侧，或屈曲的食指第一指间关节骨突部点压受术体表。

Ⅱ．Requirements

Thumb pointing manipulation is to use the thumb tip to press the therapeutic region; inflectional-finger point manipulation is to use the radial side of the inflectional interphalangeal joints of the thumb or the apophysis of the first interphalangeal joints of the inflectional index finger to press the therapeutic region.

三、注意事项

本法刺激性强，使用时要根据病人的具体情况和操作部位酌情用力。用力宜平稳，一般不要冲击用力。

Ⅲ．Notes

Because of strong irritation, using this manipulation should depend on patients' specific conditions and operation region. The force should be steady. Generally do not exert the strength suddenly.

四、临床应用

本法具有开通闭塞、活血止痛、调整脏腑功能的作用。常用于肌肉较薄的骨缝处，脘腹挛痛、腰腿痛等病证常用本法治疗。

Ⅳ. Clinical Application

Clinically, using this manipulation has functions to open the occlusion part of the body, activate blood, alleviate pain and adjust the function of visceral organs. It is applicable to bone joints where the muscles are thinner and it is commonly used to treat abdominal spasm and pain and lumbocrural pain, etc.

第十一节　捏　法
Section Eleven   Pinching Manipulation

一、概念

以手指相对用力挤压肢体,称为捏法。捏法分为二指捏、三指捏和五指捏等。

Ⅰ. Definition

This manipulation refers to squeezing the therapeutic region with fingers. It can be divided into double finger pinching manipulation, three-finger pinching manipulation and five-finger pinching manipulation, etc.

二、动作要领

以拇指与食指或食中两指夹住肢体,或五指夹住肢体,相对用力挤压。

Ⅱ. Requirements

Use the thumb and index finger (or the index and middle finger) or five fingers to clamp the body and squeeze the therapeutic region.

三、注意事项

挤压动作要均匀而有节律性。

Ⅲ. Notes

Squeezing should be uniform and rhythmic.

四、临床应用

本法具有舒筋活络、行气活血的作用,适用于颈项部、头部、四肢及脊背。

Ⅳ. Clinical Application

Clinically, using this manipulation has functions to relax the muscles and tendons and promote flow of qi and blood circulation. It is applicable to neck, head, arms, legs and back.

第十二节　拿　法
Section Twelve　Grasping Manipulation

一、概念

捏而提起谓之拿。拿法分为三指拿和五指拿法。

Ⅰ. Definition

Grasping manipulation is the combination of pinching and lifting. It can be divided into three-finger grasping manipulation and five-finger grasping manipulation.

二、动作要领

以拇指与食中两指，或用拇指与其余四指相对用力，在受术部位或穴位上作节律性地提捏。

Ⅱ. Requirements

Use the thumb, the index and the middle finger or the thumb and the other four fingers to hold and squeeze the therapeutic region or acupoints rhythmically.

三、注意事项

要指面着力，不要以指端抓抠；提拿时腕关节要放松灵活，略作掌屈；用力要由轻到重，再由重到轻，不可突发用力；动作宜缓和而有连贯性。临床上常与揉法结合运用。

Ⅲ. Notes

Use the finger cushion instead of the fingertip. When grasping, wrist joints should be relaxed and keep palmar flexion slightly. Exert the strength from light to heavy, and then from heavy to light. Don't exert the strength suddenly. The action should be mitigative and consistent. Clinically, it is usually combined with kneading manipulation.

四、临床应用

具有祛风散寒、舒筋通络等作用。常配合其他手法运用于项部、肩部和四肢等部位，如拿项部、拿肩井、拿三角肌、拿承山、拿肚角等。通常用于治疗头痛、项强、四肢关节及肌肉酸痛等病证。

Ⅳ. Clinical Application

Clinically, using this manipulation has functions to expel wind and cold and relax the muscles and tendons. It is applicable to napex, shoulder, arms and legs in combination with other manipulations, such as grasping napex, grasping Jianjing (GB 21), grasping deltoid, grasping Chengshan (BL 57), and grasping Dujiao, and so on. It is commonly used to treat headache, cervical rigidity, ache in limbs and muscles, etc.

第十三节　捻　法
Section Thirteen　Holding-twisting Manipulation

一、概念

拇食二指捏住肢体作快速搓动，称为捻法。

Ⅰ. Definition

The manipulation refers to twisting some parts fast with the thumb and index finger.

二、动作要领

用拇指指纹面与屈曲的食指中节桡侧，或伸直的食指末节指纹面捏住手指或脚趾，相对作快速搓动。

Ⅱ. Requirements

Use the surface of thumb and the radial side of the middle part of the inflectional index finger or the surface of the end of the straight index finger. Hold fingers or toes, and then twist them rapidly.

三、注意事项

搓动灵活、快速，用劲不可呆滞；着力是一个面，而不是一个点。本法作用到皮下组织和肌肉,不可与受术者皮肤发生摩擦。捻手指时可边捻边移动。

Ⅲ. Notes

Twist fast and flexibly but not dully. The force should be applied in a region instead of a point. This manipulation affects subcutaneous tissues and muscles, so it cannot have friction with patients' skin. Holding and twisting fingers can combine with moving.

四、临床应用

本法一般适用于手指和脚趾,具有理筋活络、滑利关节的作用,常配合其他手法治疗指(趾)间关节的酸痛、肿胀或屈伸不利等症。

Ⅳ. Clinical Application

Clinically, this manipulation is applicable to fingers and toes and have functions to relax the muscles and tendons and lubricate joints. It is commonly used to treat symptoms of aching pain, swelling, inconvenient flexing and stretching of finger and toe joints, etc.

第十四节 抖 法
Section Fourteen　Shaking Manipulation

一、概念

将患者的四肢作连续、小幅度的快速抖动,称为抖法。

Ⅰ. Definition

Shaking the patient's limbs in a continuous, rapid and small-extent way is called shaking manipulation

二、动作要领

用双手握住患者的上肢或下肢远端,用力作连续、小幅度地上下或左右抖动。

Ⅱ. Requirements

Hold the distal end of the patient's upper limbs or lower limbs by two hands and shake up and down or left and right to a small extent by power.

三、注意事项

操作时抖动幅度要小,频率要快。抖上肢也可单手操作。

Ⅲ. Notes

The shaking extent should be small while the frequency should be high when manipulating. The upper limbs can also be shaked by one hand.

四、临床应用

本法主要有舒筋解痉作用,可用于四肢部,而以上肢为常用。常配合搓法作为治疗的结束手法。治疗作用与搓法同。

Ⅳ. Clinical Application

The clinical use of this method can relieve spasmolysis and relax muscles as well as tendons. It can be used on four limbs, especially upper limbs. Usually, it is often used as an ending manipulaton.

第十五节 振 法
Section Fifteen Vibrating Manipulation

一、概念

分为掌振法和指振法两种。

Ⅰ. Definition

It is divided into palm vibrating manipulation and finger vibrating manipulation.

二、动作要领

用手掌或手指着力于受术体表,前臂和手部的肌肉强力地静止性用力,产生较高频率的持续性振颤动作。振法的频率可达每分钟 600 次左右,掌振法的频率比指振法高。

Ⅱ. Requirements

Apply the power of your palms or fingers to the surface of the patient and exert static power, which produce highly frequent and continuous thumping action. The frequency of thumping manipulation can reach to 600 times per minute. The frequency of palm vibrating manipulation is higher than that of finger vibrating manipulation by finger.

三、注意事项

振法的振动方向应与受术体表相垂直,不要横向振动。振法的垂直压力不可太大。操作者自然呼吸,不可屏气。为使本法维持足够的操作时间,手臂屈肌和伸肌的收缩与放松要协调。

Ⅲ. Notes

The direction of vibrating manipulation should be perpendicular to the patient's surface. The direction can't be left and right. The perpendicular force of vibrating manipulation can't be too large. The manipulator should breathe naturally rather than hold his or her breath. In order to keep manipulating for a time, the contraction of the flexor and extensor muscles should harmonize with the relaxation of the flexor and extensor muscles.

四、临床应用

本法具有解痉镇痛、宣肺化痰、补气益肾、健脾和胃等作用,一般常用单手操作。

Ⅳ. Clinical Application

This method can relieve spasmolysis and analgesia, ventilate the lung and resolve phlegm, reinforce qi, tonify kidney, and strengthen the spleen and stomach. Basically, we use one-hand manipulation.

第十六节　拍　法
Section Sixteen　Patting Manipulation

一、概念

用手掌拍打体表,称拍法。

Ⅰ. Definition

The manipulation of patting the body surface by palm is called patting manipulation.

二、动作要领

五指自然并拢,掌指关节微屈,以虚掌平稳而有节奏地拍打患部。

Ⅱ. Requirements

The five fingers draw close to each other naturally with metacarpophalangeal joints lightly flexed to pat the affected region by empty palm steadily and rhythmically.

三、注意事项

要以虚掌拍打,手掌周围一圈同时接触,手指不要甩动,以免造成病人痛苦。以肘带臂,以臂带腕,以腕带掌。可单手拍打,也可双手交替拍击。对于面积较小的受术部位(如面部),掌拍法可改为三指拍法。

Ⅲ. Notes

Pat with empty palm. The circle around the palm should touch the affected region at the same time and the fingers should avoid switching for fear of causing pain on patients. Drive the arm with the elbow, drive the wrist with the arm, and drive the palm with the wrist. Pat by one hand or pat by alternate hands. For body surface of small area (such as face), patting with the palm is better than that with three fingers.

四、临床应用

具有舒筋活络、行气活血、宣肺化痰等作用。拍法常用于肩背、腰臀及下肢部。对风湿酸痛、局部感觉迟钝、麻木或肌肉痉挛、咳喘痰多等症常用本法配合其他手法治疗。

Ⅳ. Clinical Application

This manipulation has clinical effects on relaxing tendons, activating collaterals, promoting qi, activating blood circulation, ventilating the lung and resolving phlegm and so on. Patting manipulation is commonly applied on shoulder, back, waist, buttock, and lower limbs. For treating rheumatic pain, localized dysesthesia, numbness or muscle spasm, cough and asthma with excessive phlegm and other syndromes, patting manipulation can cooperate with other manipulations.

第十七节 击 法
Section Seventeen Hitting Manipulation

一、概念

用拳背、掌根、掌侧小鱼际、指尖或桑枝棒叩击体表，称击法。

Ⅰ. Definition

Using the back of fist, the root of the palm, the minor thenar eminence, the fingertip or a stick made of mulberry twig to beat the surface of the body is called hitting manipulation.

二、动作要领

（1）拳背击法是手握空拳、腕关节挺直，用拳背平击体表。

（2）掌根击法是手指自然松开、腕伸直，用掌根部叩击体表。

（3）侧击法（又称小鱼际击）是手指自然伸直、腕略背伸，用单手或双手小鱼际部击打体表。

（4）指尖击法是用指端轻轻击打体表，如雨点下落。

（5）棒击法是用桑枝棒击打体表。

Ⅱ. Requirements

（1）Fist-back hitting: The operating hand should turn into empty fist and his wrist joint should be straightened. The back of fist should be used to beat surface of the body.

（2）Palm-root tapping: The fingers of the operating hand should be loosened naturally with straight wrist. The root of the palm should be used to beat surface of the body.

（3）Side-hitting（minor thenar eminence-hitting）: The finger of the operating hand should be naturally straight and the wrist should be slightly dorsal stretch. The ulnar surface of minor thenar eminence of one or two hands can be used to beat surface of the body.

（4）Fingertip hitting: The tip of the fingers should hit the surface of the body as gently as the rain falling.

（5）Stick striking: It is a manipulation by using stick made of mulberry twig to hit the surface of the body.

三、注意事项

用力要快速而短暂；用力的方向要与体表垂直，不能有拖抽动作；速度要均匀而有节奏；击打肌肉丰厚处，避开骨骼突起部；棒击四肢时棒的方向要与肢体纵轴平行，不可施横棒；击打头顶时用力宜轻。

Ⅲ. Notes

The force in the manipulation should be quick and brief. The direction of the force should be perpendicular to the surface of the body without dragging. The velocity should be even and rhythmed. Thick muscles can be hit, but the protuberance of the bones should be avoided. When you do the stick striking, the stick should be parallel to the vertical axis of the limbs. You should hit the head slightly.

四、临床应用

本法具有舒筋活络、调和气血之功，对风湿痹痛、感觉迟钝等症常用本法配合治疗。拳背击法常用于腰背部；掌根击法常用于头顶、腰臀及四肢部；侧击法常用于腰背及四肢部；指尖法常用于头面、胸腹部；棒击法常用于头顶、腰背及四肢部。

Ⅳ. Clinical Application

This manipulation has the effects on relaxing muscles and tendons and activating the flow of qi and blood. It can usually applied in rheumatism pain, dysesthesia and so on. Fist-back hitting is mainly applied to lower back. Palm-root tapping is mainly applied to the top of the head, waist, hip and limps. Side-hitting is usually applied to low back and limbs. Fingertip hitting is always suitable for the head, face, chest and abdomen. Stick striking is mainly suitable for the top of the head, the low back and limbs.

第十八节 弹 法
Section Eighteen Flicking Manipulation

一、概念

以手指的指甲弹击受术部位，称为弹法。

Ⅰ. Definition

Using the nail of the finger to flick the body is called flicking manpulation.

二、动作要领

手握空拳，拇指指腹紧扣住中指(或食指)的指甲，中指(或食指)由屈曲位置从拇指指腹突然滑脱而伸直，以指甲部着力连续弹击受术部位，频率为每分钟 120—160 次。

Ⅱ. Requirements

The operating hand should turn into a empty fist. The finger pulp of thumb should buckle the nail of the middle finger or index finger. The middle finger or the index finger suddenly slips and changes the flexed position to the extending position to flick the body continually by the nail. You should flick it 120 – 160 times per minute.

三、注意事项

用力适中，要有一定的节律。本法还可以由中指扣住食指，以食指指甲用力弹击。

Ⅲ. Notes

The force of the manipulation should be appropriate and rhythmed. This manipulation can also be applied by middle finger and index finger. The middle finger should buckle the nail of index finger and the nail of the index finger can be applied to flick hard.

四、临床应用

本法具有舒筋活络、疏风散寒的作用。适用于全身各部，尤以头面、颈项部最为常用，对外感头痛、项强、失眠等症，常用本法配合治疗。

Ⅳ. Clinical Application

This manipulation has the effects on relaxing muscles and tendons and treats the cold. It is mainly applied to the whole body, especially for the head, face and neck. When you treat exogenous headache, cervical rigidity, insomnia and so on, this manipulation can be used.

第十九节 摇 法
Section Nineteen Rotating Manipulation

一、概念

使关节作被动的环转活动，称摇法。

Ⅰ. Definition

Making the joint to do the passive circumduction is called rotating manipulation.

二、动作要领

（1）颈项部摇法：用一手扶住患者头顶后部（或托住患者枕部），另一手托住下颌，双手协调作颈椎环转摇动。

（2）肩关节摇法：用一手扶住患者肩部，另一手握住腕部或托住肘部，作肩部环转运动。

（3）髋关节摇法：患者仰卧位，髋膝屈曲。术者一手托住患者足跟，另一手扶住膝部，作髋关节环转摇动。

（4）踝关节摇法：用一手托住患者足跟，另一手握住足尖部，作踝关节环转摇动。

Ⅱ. Requirements

（1）The rotating of the neck: Use one hand to hold the patient's head back or occipitalis and the other hand to hold the mandible. Both of the hands coordinate to make the cervical vertebra do circumduction.

（2）Shoulder rotating manipulation: Support the patient's shoulder with one hand, hold the wrist or elbow with the other, and move them orbiting the shoulder joint.

（3）Coxa rotating manipulation: Let the patient lie on his back and buckle his knee. Hold the patient's heel, knee and orbit the leg around the hip joint.

（4）Ankle shaking manipulation: Hold the patient's heel and tiptoes with the other and shake the foot around the ankle.

三、注意事项

摇法动作要缓和，用力要稳。摇动幅度须在患者生理许可范围内，由小到大操作。

Ⅲ. Notes

The manipulation should be soft and stable. The range of movement should be based on the patient's condition, and start from the mild action.

四、临床应用

本法具有滑利关节、增强关节活动功能的作用。适用于四肢关节及颈项、腰等部位，主治关节强硬、屈伸不利等症。

IV. Clinical Application

The manipulation can lubricate and strengthen joints in clinical use. It can be applied on joints of arms, legs, neck, waist, etc. The manipulation indicates syndromes like anchylosis, inhibited bending and stretching.

第二十节 背 法
Section Twenty   Back-packing Manipulation

一、概念

将患者反背起，利用自身重量牵引脊柱，并作抖晃动作，称为背法。

I. Definition

Back-packing manipulation is to carry the patient on your back, shake his body and tract the spine with the help of gravity.

二、动作要领

术者和患者背靠背站立，术者两肘套住患者肘弯部，然后弯腰屈膝挺臀，将患者反背起，使其双脚离地，利用自身重量牵伸脊柱片刻；以尾骶部着力抵住患者腰部，使患者腰以下随之作左右摆动；再作快速伸膝挺臀动作，以加强腰部牵引的效果，或使错位的小关节得以整复。

II. Requirements

The doctor and the patient should stand back to back and elbows hooking elbows, and then the doctor raises the patient until his feet leaves the ground; use coccygeal bodies to move the patient's lower part, extend the hip and knee to strengthen the waist and repair the moved tiny joints.

三、注意事项

嘱患者全身放松，头颈部靠住术者背部；年老体弱、骨质疏松者慎用。

III. Notes

The patient should relax and stick his neck to the doctor's back. It should be careful applied to the weak, the old and those with osteoporosis.

四、临床应用

本法可使腰脊柱伸展,使扭错之小关节易于复位,并有助于缓解腰痛症状。适用于腰部扭闪疼痛、腰椎退行性脊柱炎等病证。

Ⅳ. Clinical Application

Clinically the manipulation can extend spine to repair the moved joints and alleviate the waist pain. This manipulation is suitable to lumbar sprain or degenerative diseases, etc.

第二十一节　扳　法
Section Twenty-one　Pulling Manipulation

一、概念

用双手向相反方向或同一方向用力扳动肢体称为扳法。

Ⅰ. Definition

Pulling manipulation is to use hands to pull body in the same direction or the opposite.

二、动作要领

1. 颈项部扳法

常用方法为颈部旋转定位扳法。患者坐位,术者站于其后,用一肘部托住其下颌部,手则扶住其枕部,使患者颈前屈到某一需要的角度后,另一手扶住患者肩部,托起头部得手用力,先作颈项部向上牵引,同时把患者头部作被动向患侧旋转至最大限度后,再作扳法。

2. 胸背部扳法

常用的有两种扳法。

第一种为扩胸牵引扳法,患者坐位,另其双手交叉扣住,置于项部。术者两手托住患者两肘部,并用一侧膝部顶住患者背部,嘱患者自行俯仰,并配合深呼吸,作扩胸牵引扳动。

第二种为胸椎对抗复位法,患者坐位,另其双手交叉扣住,置于项部。术者在其后面,用两手从患者腋部伸入其上臂之前,前臂之后,并握住其前臂下段,同时术者用一膝部顶住患部脊椎,嘱患者身体略向前倾,术者两手同时作向后上方用力扳动。

3. 腰部扳法

常用的有两种扳法。

第一种为斜扳法,患者侧卧位,术者用一手抵住患者肩前部,另一手抵住臀部,或一手抵住患者肩后部另一手抵住髂前上棘部。把腰被动旋转至最大限度后,两手同时作相反方向扳动。

第二种为腰部旋转扳法,此法又有三种方法。其一为直腰旋转扳法。患者坐位,术者用腿夹住患者下肢,一手抵住患者近术者侧的肩后部,另一手从患者腋下伸入抵住肩前部,两手同时用力作相反方向扳动。其二为弯腰旋转扳法。患者坐位,腰前屈到某一需要角度后,一助手帮助固定患者下肢及骨盆,术者以一手拇指按住需扳动的脊椎的棘突(向左旋转时用右手),另一手勾扶住患者项背部(向左旋转时用左手),使其腰部在前屈位时再向患侧旋转,至最大限度时,再使其腰部向健侧侧弯方向扳动。其三为腰部后伸扳法。患者俯卧位,术者一手托住患者两膝部,缓缓向上提起,另一手紧压在腰部患处,当腰后伸到最大限度时,两手同时用力作相反方向扳动。

Ⅱ. Requirements

1. Neck Pulling Manipulation

Neck pulling manipulation is the commonly-used one. The patient should sit in front of the doctor and the doctor should hold his jaw and head back with hands. Move the neck to some extend and hold his shoulder with one hand and pull and rotate the neck to the maximum before pulling.

2. Chest and Back Pulling Manipulation

There are two common pulling manipulation.

One is chest-expanding and tracting manipulation. The patient should take a seat and cross arms in front of chest. The doctor holds the patient's elbows and supports his back with a knee to ask the patient to pitch corresponding to breath.

The other is chest spinal conflict recovery manipulation. The patient sits down and crosses his arms above head. The doctor stands at the back and handles the front arm through the patient's axilla and supports his back with a knee to ask the patient to lean forward and extend upwards with hands from the back.

3. Pulling Manipulation on Waist

There are two common pulling manipulation.

The first one is oblique pulling manipulation. The surgeon use one hand against the patient's front shoulder and the other hand against the hip or hand against patient's back and the other hand against the anterior superior iliac spine portion. Shift the patient's waist to the furthest and pull with two hands.

The second one is rotating pulling manipulation on waist. It has three modes. The first one is to pull with waist straight. The patient should take a seat, and the surgeon catches patient's lower limb with legs, with one hand against the shoulder near the surgeon and another hand crossing the patient's armpit against the front portion of shoulder; pull the patient's waist with two hands. The second one is to pull with waist bent. The patient should take a seat and bend the waist to the front to a required angle. An assistant helps to fix the patient's lower extremities and pelvis. Surgeon uses one thumb against the requested spine spinous process (use right hand when rotating to the left). The other hand hooks patient's nape (use left hand when rotating to the left), makes the waist rotating to the affected side in anterior flexion to the furthest; pull the waist to the uninjured side. The third one is to pull while waist extending. The patient takes prone position. Surgeon use one hand to hold the patient's two knees, and rises the knees slowly with one hand, presses the injured waist tightly with the other hand. When the waist extends to the furthest, pulling with two hands.

三、注意事项

扳法操作时动作必须果断而快速,用力要稳,两手动作配合要协调。扳动幅度一般不能超过各关节的生理活动范围。

Ⅲ. Notes

When pulling, the surgeon must be fast, stable and coordinately with two hands. The range should be within the physiological range of the joints motions.

四、临床应用

本法具有舒筋活络、滑利关节、纠正解剖位置的异常等作用,临床常与其他手法配合应用。多用于脊柱及四肢关节的错位或关节功能障碍等症。

Ⅳ. Clinical Application

Pulling manipulation can simulate the circulation of the blood and relax the muscles and joints and correct anatomical location of abnormalities. It often coordinates other manipulation and applys to spine and limbs joint dislocation or joint dysfunction embolism.

第二十二节　拔伸法
Section Twenty-two　Tracting-countertracting Manipulation

一、概念

拔伸即牵拉的意思。固定肢体或关节的一端,牵拉另一端的方法称为拔伸法。

Ⅰ. Definition

This method means fixing one end of a limb or joint, and then pull the other end.

二、动作要领

头项部拔伸法:患者正坐,术者站于患者背后,用双手拇指顶在枕骨下方,掌根托住两侧下颌角的下方,并用两前臂压住患者两肩,两手用力向上,两前臂下压,同时作相反方向用力。

肩关节拔伸法:患者坐位,术者用双手握住其腕部或肘部,逐渐用力牵拉,嘱患者身体向另一侧倾斜,与牵拉之力对抗。

腕关节拔伸法:术者一手握住患者前臂下端,另一手握住其手部,两手同时向相反方向用力,逐渐牵拉。

指间关节拔伸法:用一手捏住被拔伸关节的近侧端,另一手捏住其远侧端,两手同时向相反方向用力牵引。

Ⅱ. Requirements

Tracting manipulation of head: Asking the patient to sit, the practitioner stands behind the patient. Use two thumbs to press below the occipital. Hold the bottom of the mandibular angle both sides with the heel of the hand. And press the patient's shoulders with forearms with hands forcibly upward and forearms pushing down in the opposite direction.

Tracting manipulation of shoulder joint: The patient is in a sitting position. The practitioner holds the patient's wrists or elbows with both hands and then pulls gradually, asking the patient to lean his body towards the other side against the force of pulling.

Tracting manipulation of wrist joint: The practitioner uses one hand to hold the patient's lower part of his forearm and the other hand to hold his hand. Then the practitioner's two hands simultaneously apply the opposing forces and then pull gradually.

Tracting manipulation of interphalangeal joint: hold the proximal end of the injured joint with one hand and the distal end with the other. Then the practitioner's two hands simultaneously apply the opposing forces and then pull forcibly.

三、注意事项

本法操作时用力要均匀而持久,动作要缓和。

Ⅲ. Notes

The strength should be equal and long; the operation should be moderate.

四、临床应用

本法常用于关节错位伤筋等,对扭错的肌腱和移位的关节有整复作用。

Ⅳ. Clinical Application

Tracting-countertracting manipulation is used to correct joints dislocation and others; and has the reduction effect on twisted tendons and dislocated joints.

第二十三节　小儿推拿常用手法
Section Twenty-three　Commonly-used Infantile Tuina Manipulations

小儿推拿手法是与成人推拿手法相对而言的。大多数小儿推拿手法是与成人手法类似或通用的,只是在手法的运用上更为符合小儿的解剖特点和生理、病理特点而已。只有个别手法只适用于小儿而不用于成人,如运法。

小儿推拿手法在成人推拿手法的基本要求的基础上,特别强调轻快柔和、平稳着实。根据病情的轻重和患儿年龄的大小,在手法操作次数或时间上有明显的区别。一般来说,年龄大、病情重者,操作次数多、时间长;年龄小、病情轻者,操作次数少、时间短。

Infantile tuina manipulation is referred compared with adult tuina one; most of the former are similar to the latter, or are shared in use with the latter. Though its application more conforms to the anatomical, physiological and pathological characteristics of children. Only a few manipulation methods are only suitable for children, such as *yun* method.

Infantile tuina emphasizes lightness, softness and steadiness on the basis of the basic requirements of adult tuina. According to the state of an illness and the patient' age，manipulation times or time differ significantly. In general，older-aged cases or those in severe conditions will receive more manipulations for longer time，and *vice versa*.

一、推法

1. 概念
小儿推拿的推法包括直推、旋推、分推、合推四种。

2. 动作要领
直推法是用拇指绕侧缘或指纹面，或食中二指指纹面作单方向的直线推动。旋推法是用右手拇指指纹面在穴位上作顺时针方向的旋转摩动，一般不带动皮下组织。分推法是用双手拇指桡侧缘或指纹面，自受术部位的中点向两旁作分离推动，一般为直线运动，也可走弧线。合法是用双手拇指指纹面从穴位两旁向中间推动。

3. 临床应用
直推法是小儿推拿的常用手法，适用于线状部位，如开天门、推天柱骨、推大肠、推三关等。旋推法主要用于手部面状穴位，如旋推脾经、肺经、肾经等。分推法适用于坎宫、大横纹、腹、肺俞等。合推法临床应用较少，仅用于合推大横纹。

Ⅰ. Pushing Manipulation

1. Definition
The pushing manipulation of infantile tuina includes direct pushing，whirly pushing，apart pushing and combined pushing.

2. Requirements
Direct pushing means that pushing along the edge or fingerprint surface of the thumb，or the fingerprint surface of the middle finger in the unidirectional straight direction. Whirly pushing means that using the fingerprint surface of the right thumb to rotate clockwise on the acupuncture point，without affecting the subcutaneous tissues. Apart pushing means that using the radial lateral margin or fingerprint surface of the thumbs to do pushing outwards from the center of the manipulated parts generally in straight motion and sometimes arched motion. Combined pushing means that using the fingerprint surface of the thumbs to push from the sides of acupoints to its middle.

3. Clinical Application
Direct pushing is the commonly-used infantile tuina technique，appropriate for the linear parts，like "Open Tian Men"，"Push Tianzhu Bone"，"Push Large Intestine"，"Push Triple Guan". Whirly pushing is mainly used in the planar acupoints on hands，such as whirly pushing spleen channel，lung channel and kidney channel. Apart

pushing can be used in Kangong, Dahengwen, the abdomen and Feishu. Combined pushing is rarely used in the clinical application, but in pushing Dahengwen.

二、揉法

1. 概念

揉法分掌揉和指揉两种。掌揉法包括鱼际揉和掌根揉;指揉法包括一指揉、二指揉、三指揉等。

2. 动作要领

用手掌鱼际、掌根部分或手指指纹面部分,吸定于受术者部位或穴位上,作轻柔缓和回旋揉动。指揉中多用拇指或中指指纹面操作,称单指揉;用食、中指同揉一处或分揉二穴者,称双指揉;用食、中、无名三指同揉一处或分揉三穴者,称为三指揉。

3. 临床应用

本法具有宽胸理气、消积导滞、活血祛瘀、消肿止痛作用。揉法轻柔缓和、刺激量小,适用于全身各部。二指揉可用于同时揉睛明等对称性穴位。三指揉适用于同时指揉神阙和两侧天枢,常用于脘腹胀通、胸闷胁痛、便秘及泄泻等肠胃道疾患,以及因外伤引起的红肿疼痛等症。

Ⅱ. Kneading Manipulation

1. Definition

Kneading manipulation is divided into palm-kneading and finger-kneading. Palm-kneading includes Yuji (LU10) kneading and kneading by heel of hand. Finger-kneading includes one-finger-kneading, two-finger-kneading, three-finger-kneading and so on.

2. Requirements

Put your Yuji or heel of hand or the fingerprint surface of fingers on the affected parts or acupoints. Then knead gently and slowly in circles. Finger-kneading always uses the thumb or the fingerprint surface of the middle finger, with which the manipulation is called single-finger-kneading; using the thumb and middle finger to knead one acupoint simultaneously or two acupoints respectively is called double-finger-kneading; using the the thumb, middle finger and the third finger to knead one acupoint simultaneously or knead three acupoints respectively is called triple-finger-kneading.

3. Clinical Application

This manipulation can regulate qi in the chest, promote digestion and stimulate blood circulation to end stasis, and relieve swelling and pain. Kneading manipulation, gentle and slow with light stimulation, is appropriate for the entire body. Double-finger-kneading can be simultaneously used in some symmetrical acupoints, like

Jingming（BL1）；triple-finger-kneading，simultaneously in Shenque（CV8）and Tianshu（ST 25）. This manipulation often cures abdominal distension，tight chest and hypochondriac pain，constipation/diarrhea and other gastrointestinal disorders，and trauma-induced swelling and pain.

三、按法

1. 概念

按法是用手指或手掌按压受术部位或穴位，按而留之。

2. 动作要领

拇指按法：握拳，并伸直拇指，用拇指指纹面按压。中指按法：伸直中指，用中指指端按压。掌按：腕关节背伸，用单手掌心按压。

3. 临床应用

指按适用于全身穴位，如按丰隆、按揉脊柱。中指按天突时应随小儿呼吸出入，以豁痰、催吐、利尿。掌按常用于胸背。

Ⅲ. Pressing manipulation

1. Definition

This method means using fingers or palms to press the affected part or acupoint and then retain.

2. Requirements

Press by the thumb: Clench fist，unbend the thumb and press by the fingerprint surface. Press by the middle finger: unbend the middle finger，press by the fingerprint surface. Press by palm: with wrist joint dorsal extension，press by the center of one palm.

3. Clinical application

Thumb-pressing is appropriate for acupuncture points all over the body，like pressing Fenglong（ST40），pressing and kneading spines. Pressing Tiantu（CV22）with the middle finger should cooperate with the child's breathing for eliminating phlegm，promote emesis and diuresis. Palm-pressing is often used on the chest and back.

四、掐法

1. 概念

用拇指指甲或拇、食指指甲切按穴位，称为掐法。

2. 动作要领

手握空拳，拇指伸直，紧贴于食指桡侧缘。用拇指甲垂直用力切按，不得抠动而掐破皮肤。

3. 临床应用

掐法是强刺激手法之一，常用于点状穴位，为"以指代针"之法，如掐人中、掐十王、掐老龙。主要用于开窍镇惊熄风,治疗惊风抽搐。应用时应使病儿感到疼痛,大声哭叫即止。掐后常继用拇指揉法,以减缓不适。

Ⅳ. Finger-nail Pressing Manipulation

1. Definition

This method means pressing the acupoint with the nail of the thumb or nails of the thumb and index finger.

2. Requirements

Clench fist while the thumb unbends, close to the radial side of the index finger. Pressing vertically the acupoint forcibly with the nail of the thumb. Digging is not allowed to avoid skin damage.

3. Clinical Application

Finger-nail pressing manipulation is one of the manipulations with strong stimulation, often used in punctate acupoints. So it is also known as the manipulation of replacing fingers with needles. For example, we often use it to press Renzhong, Shiwang, Laolong. It is often used for inducing resuscitation, relieving convulsion and relieving dizziness to treat epilepsy. Don't stop pressing until ill children feel pain and cry. The finger-nail pressing is often followed by the kneading manipulation to relieve the discomfort.

五、捏法

1. 概念

拇、食、中三手指相对用力挟持肌肤,称为捏法。

2. 动作要领

小儿推拿中捏法多用于捏脊,是用拇指桡侧缘顶住皮肤,食、中二指前按,三指同时用力提拿肌肤,双手交替捻动向前推行;或用食指屈曲,用食指中节桡侧缘顶住皮肤,拇指前按,二指同力提拿肌肤,双手交替捻动向前推行。捏拿肌肤不宜过多,但也不宜过少。过多则不宜向前推动,过少则皮肤交痛且容易滑脱。捏拿时不要拧转肌肤。操作时,当先捏肌肤,次提拿、次捻动、次推动,动作当协调。捏脊时通常是由下向上而行,先捏脊3遍,第4遍时要行捏三提一法,即每捏3次,向上提拿1次。

3. 临床应用

小儿捏法主要用于脊柱骨穴,故称为捏脊。又因主治疳积,所以又称为捏积。该法具有强健身体和防止多种病证的作用,已被广泛运用于小儿的治疗与保健。

Ⅴ. Pinching Manipulation

1. Definition

This method means holding the skin forcibly with the thumb, index finger and middle finger.

2. Requirements

In infantile tuina, pinching manipulation is often used in spinal pinching. With the radial side of the thumb against skin, as the index finger and middle finger press forward and the three fingers simultaneously lift & pull skin, the two hands push forward alternately in a twirling way. There is another method of pinching manipulation: With the index finger flexion and the radial side of the second joint of the index finger against skin, as the thumb presses forward and the two fingers simultaneously lift & pull skin, the two hands push forward alternately in a twirling way. The area of lifted skin should be appropriate because too much can cause the difficulty in moving forward and the opposite situation can cause pain and the difficulty of lifting skin. Twisting skin is not allowed. When using the manipulation, the procedures should be coordinated: First, pinch the skin, lift it, then entwist and finally push it. Spinal pinching is usually practiced up-down for three times; at the fourth, every three pinching requires one lifting of the skin.

3. Clinical Application

Pinching manipulation in infantile tuina is usually used in acupoints in the spinal area, so it is also called spinal pinching. And because the major function is to cure malnutrition, so it is also called chiropractic. This manipulation can improve people's health and prevent many kinds of diseases, so it has been widely used in infantile care and healthcare.

六、运法

1. 概念
用手指作弧形或环形推动,称为运法。

2. 动作要领
用拇指或中指指纹面,由此穴向彼穴或在穴周作弧形或环形推动。用力宜轻不宜重,不带动皮下组织。宜缓不宜急,每分钟 80—120 次。

3. 临床应用
运法多用于掌心,如运内劳宫、运土入水等。

Ⅵ. Arc-pushing Manipulation

1. Definition

This methods means using your fingers to do pushing in a arc-shaped or circular mode.

2. Requirements

Using your thumb or the fingerprint surface of the middle finger to do pushing from one acupoint to the other or around acupoints in a arc-shaped or circular mode. Force should be light, and should not affect the subcutaneous tissues. The manipulation should be slow, about $80-120$ times per minute.

3. Clinical Application

The manipulation is usually used in the centre of the palm, like arc-pushing Inner Laogong (PC8) and arc-pushing earth into water.

第八章 成人常见疾病的推拿治疗

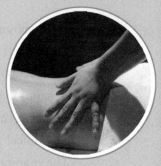

Chapter Eight Tuina Treatment for Common Diseases in Adults

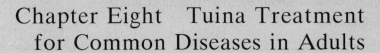

第一节 颈椎病
Section One Cervical Spondylosis

一、概念

颈椎病是指由于颈椎间盘退行性改变、颈椎骨质增生和颈部损伤等因素引起脊柱内、外平衡失调,刺激或压迫颈神经根、椎动脉、脊髓或交感神经等组织而引起的一组症状复杂、影响广泛的临床综合征,又称颈椎综合征。

本病好发于 30—60 岁人群。近年来,本病的发病率较高,有明显低龄化趋势。长期从事低头伏案工作、枕头高低或卧姿不当、颈部外伤、反复出现落枕等与本病相关。临床将颈椎病分为颈型、神经根型、椎动脉型、交感神经型、脊髓型。本病属中医的项痹病、眩晕、痿证、头痛等范畴。

Ⅰ. Definition

Cervical spondylosis is a set of clinical syndromes with complicated symptoms and signs which have wide influence, caused by degenerative discs, osteoproliferation of cervical vertebra and injury of the neck and others leading to disequilibrium of the spine and stimulation or oppression on neck nerve root, vertebral artery, spinal marrow, or sympathetic nerve and other tissues.

The disease often occurs at the age from thirty to sixty. In recent years, the incidence of the disease has been on the rise and the affected are obviously getting younger. Reasons may be as follows: bending over one's desk working for a long time, improper pillow height or sleeping posture, neck trauma, frequent neck stiffness and so on. The disease may be divided clinically into cervical type, nerve-root type, vertebral-artery type, sympathetic-nerve type and spinal-marrow type. Cervical spondylosis is categorized under "*Bi* syndrome of the neck", "dizziness syndrome", "flaccidity syndrome" and "headache" in traditional Chinese medicine.

二、病因病理

包括颈椎退行性改变、颈椎慢性损伤、颈椎急性损伤和风寒湿邪侵袭。风寒湿邪侵袭是指颈项部受风寒湿邪侵袭、经脉阻滞、肌肉痉挛致使局部组织缺血缺氧，也可出现颈椎病的一系列症状或诱发颈椎病。

Ⅱ. Etiology and Pathology

The causes includes the deterioration of cervical vertebrae, chronic injury of the neck, acute injury of the neck, and invading of wind, cold and dampness evils. Invading and attacking of wind, cold and dampness evils means that the neck and nape are attacked by the evils, leading to meridians blockage, muscle spasms and as a result, ischemia and hypoxia in local tissues and even some symptoms of cervical spondylosis or the disease.

三、临床表现

Ⅲ. Clinical Manifestation

1. 颈型颈椎病
颈型颈椎病是最早期的颈椎病，也称局部型颈椎病，其表现为：

（1）早期可见颈项、肩背部的痉挛性疼痛，颈部不敢转动或歪向一侧，转动时往往和躯干一同转动。

（2）急性期过后常常感到颈肩和上背部酸痛，不能持久伏案工作；可有头痛、后枕部疼痛和上肢无力；晨起后颈项发硬、发紧、活动不灵，反复出现"落枕"。

1. Neck Type of Cervical Spondylosis
Neck type of cervical spondylosis, the earliest stage of the disease is also called partial type of cervical spondylosis. The manifestations show as follows:

(1) In the early stage, the patient feels spastic pain in the neck, nape, shoulder and back. Because the neck can not turn towards a direction, it needs to move together with the body.

(2) After the acute period, the patient often feels aching pain in the neck, nape and upper back with headache and pain in the lateral occipitalis and weakness of upper limbs. After getting up, the patient's neck and nape may be tight and stiff with

repeated neck stiffness.

2. 神经根型颈椎病

神经根型颈椎病是中老年人的常见病,多发病。其表现为：

（1）疼痛：主要发生于头、颈项、肩背、上肢和手部,疼痛可表现为钝痛、酸痛、灼痛,或隐隐作痛,或过电样窜麻痛。

（2）麻木：麻木往往和疼痛部位相同,但麻木多出现在手指和前臂。

2. Cervical Spondylotic Radiculopathy

Cervical spondylotic radiculopathy is a common and frequently occurring disease in middle-aged and aged people. The manifestations show as follows：

（1）Pain：Pain always occurs in the head，neck and nape，shoulder and back，upper limbs and hands，including dull pain，aching pain，burning pain，and numbness & pain as if caused by electricity.

（2）Numbness：Numbness always presents where pain occurs，but more often in the fingers and forearms.

3. 椎动脉型颈椎病

椎动脉型颈椎病是由于椎动脉受压迫等而导致椎动脉供血不足的一种病证。其表现为：

（1）眩晕：常在头部转到某一方位或体位改变时,如头向上仰、突然转头或反复左右转头时发生眩晕或眩晕加重,再转回原方位时症状减轻。伴有视力减退、耳鸣、耳聋、恶心、呕吐、眼震等症状。

（2）猝倒：是椎动脉型颈椎病特有的症状,在眩晕剧烈或颈部活动时发生。

（3）头痛：呈发作性或持续性,持续数分钟或数小时,甚至数日。

（4）视觉障碍：视物模糊、复视、眼前闪光、暗点、一过性黑矇、暂时性视野缺损,甚至失明等视力障碍。

3. Vertebral Artery Type of Cervical Spondylosis

Vertebral artery type of cervical spondylosis is caused by the shortage of blood-supply to vertebral arteries which results in pressure on vertebral arteries. Its representations are as follows：

（1）Vertigo：Vertigo always occurs when the patient turns his/her head towards certain direction or changes the body position，such as raising the head. For example，turning the head suddenly or turning the head left and right repeatedly can make the vertigo worse while turning back to the original position can lessen it. Moreover，the symptom is always accompanied by hypopsia，tinnitus，deafness，nausea，vomiting，nystagmus and so on.

（2）Cataplexy：Cataplexy is a special symptom of vertebral artery type of cervical spondylosis，which occurs during severe vertigo and the activity of cervical part.

（3）Headache：Headache is paroxysmal and persistent. It can continue for several minutes or hours，and even several days.

（4）Visual disorder：blurred vision，diplopia，aethomma，scotoma，amaurosis fugax，temporary loss of vision，or even blindness and other visual disorders.

4. 交感神经型颈椎病

交感神经型颈椎病是由于颈椎退行性变,后关节增生等刺激或压迫颈部交感神经而出现的一组证候群。其表现为：

（1）眼睑无力,视物模糊,眼窝部胀痛,流泪,视野内冒金星,怕光,视力减退,瞳孔扩大或缩小。

（2）头痛或偏头痛、头晕,以及面部发热、充血、麻木等。

（3）心慌、心悸、心律不齐,心前区疼痛,阵发性心动过速,血压时高时低。

（4）血管痉挛引起肢体发凉、局部皮温下降、皮肤凉且有刺痒感,继而出现红肿或疼痛加重,或因血管扩张引起指端发热、发红、疼痛或痛觉过敏,肢体、头、颈、面部麻木。

（5）局部肢体或半侧身体多汗或少汗,皮肤发绀、发凉、干燥、变薄,毛发过多或毛发干枯、脱落,指甲干燥无光泽,以及营养性皮肤溃疡等。

（6）耳鸣、听力减退,甚至耳聋。鼻咽部不适、疼痛,鼻塞,或有异味感。咽喉部不适或发干、异物感、嗳气、牙痛、舌麻木等。

4. Sympathetic Type of Cervical Spondylosis

Sympathetic type of cervical spondylosis includes a group of syndromes caused by the degeneration of cervical vertebrae，the hyperplasia of posterior joints and other stimulation or pressure on the sympathetic nerve of the cervical part. Its presentations are as follows：

（1）Weak eyelid，blurred vision，lacrimation，sparks flew before one's eyes，fear of light，visual deterioration，mydriasis or miosis.

（2）Headache or migraine，dizziness，and facial fever，redness and numbness.

（3）Palpitations，arrhythmia，precordial pain，paroxysmal tachycardia. The blood pressure is sometimes high and sometimes low.

（4）Coldness of limbs caused by vasospasm，lower temperature of local skin，cold and itching skin followed by worse redness and pain，fever，redness，pain，or hyperalgesia of the finger tips and numbness of limbs，head，neck and face caused by vasodilatation.

（5）Local limbs or half of the body are hyperhidrotic or hypohidrotic；cyanosis，cold，drying and thining of skin；hypertrichosis，parch blight or abscission of hair；finger nails are dry and dull，dermal ulcer.

（6）Tinnitus，amblyacousia，even deafness；discomfort，pain，obstruction or foreign body sensation in pharynx nasalis，discomfort，drying and foreign body sensation in the throat，belching，toothache，numbness of the tongue and so on.

5. 脊髓型颈椎病

脊髓型颈椎病是由于颈脊髓受到压迫后引起的以肢体功能障碍为特征的一组证候

群。早期病人常出现一侧上下肢或两侧上下肢单纯的运动障碍、感觉障碍或两者同时存在，亦可为一侧上肢和对侧下肢感觉、运动障碍，所以脊髓型颈椎病的症状较为复杂。其表现为：

（1）脊髓单侧受压：临床比较少见。

（2）脊髓双侧受压：较单侧受压多见，主要表现为缓慢进行性双下肢麻木、发冷、疼痛，步态不稳、笨拙、发抖无力等。病人主诉如"踩棉花感""头重脚轻""欲倒"等。初期常呈间歇性，劳累、行走过多等可使症状加剧。少数病人偶尔可于猛烈仰头时感到全身麻木，双腿发软，甚至摔倒。随着病情发展，症状可逐渐加剧并转为持续性，表现为上运动神经元或锥体束损害不完全痉挛性瘫痪，以至卧床不起，甚至呼吸困难。

（3）另外，临床上有两型或两型以上的颈椎病证状、体征者，即可视为混合型颈椎病。混合型颈椎病在临床较为常见，其主要原因是神经根、椎动脉、交感神经纤维、颈段脊髓等组织在解剖上密切联系，当椎间盘向后侧突出时，常同时压迫两种以上的组织。因此，从解剖学和病理学上看，多种组织混合受累是绝对的，而单纯的神经根、椎动脉或脊髓受累是相对的。

5. Cervical Spondylotic Myelopathy Type

Cervical spondylotic myelopathy （CSM） includes a group of syndromes characterized by limbs dysfunction due to cervical cord compression. Patients always have paresthesia or akinesis with unilateral or bilateral upper and lower limbs or even both in the early stage. The patients can also have paresthesia or akinesis with unilateral upper limbs and contralateral lower limbs. So the symptoms of cervical spondylotic myelopathy are very complicated. Its expressions includes:

（1）Unilateral compression of spinal cord, a clinical rare presentation.

（2）Bilateral compression of spinal cord which is much more common than unilateral compression of spinal cord. The main presentations are chronic progressive anesthesia, cold and pain in the lower limbs, unsteady walk, lumbering gait, shake, weakness and so on. Patients may also complain of "feeling walking on sponge", "feeling top-heavy", "feel like falling", etc. It is intermittent in the early stage and too much work or walk will make the symptoms worse. A few patients sometimes will experience general numbness; weakness of legs, and even fall over when raising their heads suddenly. As the illness develops, the symptoms will become worse and continuous. As a result, the patient may have the presentation of incomplete spastic paralysis resulting from an upper motor neuron or pyramidal tract lesion, so that he/she will be bed-ridden and even have difficulty breathing.

（3）In addition, it will be defined as mixed-type CSM, if there are two or more kinds symptoms or signs of CSM. The mixed type is very common clinically. It will compress two or more kinds of tissues when the discus intervertebralis protrude backward because nerve root, vertebral artery, sympathetic fiber and spinal cord are closely tied up with each other in anatomy. Therefore, anatomically and pathologically, mixed involvement among a variety of tissues is absolute while the simple involvement among nerve root, vertebral artery or spinal cord is relative.

四、诊断要点

Ⅳ. Diagnostic Points

1. 颈型颈椎病

（1）颈部肌肉痉挛，肌张力增高，颈项强直，活动受限。

（2）颈项部有广泛压痛。

（3）颈椎 X 线检查：颈椎生理曲度变直、反弓或成角，有轻度的骨质增生。

1. Cervical Spondylosis of Neck Type

（1）Muscle spasm in the neck, hypermyotonia, neck rigidity and limitation of activity.

（2）General tenderness in the neck.

（30 X-ray exam: Cervical physiological curvature becomes straight, reverse or angled with mild bone hyperplasia.

2. 神经根型颈椎病

（1）手和前臂部位的感觉减退，少数有感觉过敏。病久者病变神经根支配的肌肉发生肌力减退、肌张力降低，手和上肢发冷以及肌肉萎缩。肱二头肌、肱三头肌反射和桡骨膜反射减弱或消失。

（2）椎间孔挤压试验和臂丛神经牵拉试验阳性。

（3）颈椎 X 线检查：正位片可见颈椎侧弯、钩椎关节增生、棘突偏歪等；侧位片可见颈椎生理曲度变直、成角、反弓，椎间隙狭窄、椎体移位、椎体后缘增生、椎体前缘增生过大可形成骨桥、项韧带钙化等。

2. Cervical Spondylotic Radiculopathy Type

（1）Hypoesthesia in the hand and forearm and hyperaesthesia in some will occur. For the patient affected by the disease for a long time, the muscle controlled by diseased nerve roots will present diminished strength and muscular tension; cold in the hand and upper limbs, amyotrophy; and decreased or disappeared bicipital reflex, triceps reflex and radioperiosteal reflex.

（2）The cervical foraminal compression test and brachial plexus traction test show positive.

（3）X-ray exam: Cervical vertebra scoliosis, hyperplasia of uncovertebral joint , setover of crest can be found in the anterioposterior film. Straight, reverse or angled cervical physiological curvature, narrowing of vertebrae and disc, shift of centrums, hyperplasia of centrums posterior border，bone bridge formed in centrums posterior border and ligamentum nuchae ossification can be found in the lateral film.

3. 椎动脉型颈椎病

（1）后枕部触诊检查：患者棘突多有病理性移位，相应的关节囊部位肿胀、压痛。

（2）患者作颈部较大幅度的旋转、后伸活动时，可引起突然眩晕、四肢麻木、软弱无力而猝倒。

（3）旋颈试验阳性。

（4）经颅多普勒超声检查：椎-基底动脉血流速度降低，脑血流量减少（一部分为椎-基底动脉痉挛，流速加快）。

3. Cervical Spondylosis of Vertebral Artery Type

（1）Palpation of the occipital: There is always a pathologic shift on the spinous process of patients; swelling and tenderness are felt in the corresponding parts of the articular capsule.

（2）Relatively drastic neck rotation and backward extension activities for the patient can cause sudden dizziness, numbness and weakness of the limbs and then cataplexy.

（3）The neck rotation test (Revolve-cervix test) shows positive.

（4）Transcranial Doppler ultrasound (TCD): Blood flow velocity is reduced in vertebrobasilar artery, and cerebral blood flow is diminished (Spasms occur in some vertebrobasilar arteries resulting in increased flow velocity).

4. 交感神经型颈椎病

（1）颈部肌肉痉挛、活动障碍及棘突旁有压痛、棘突或横突偏移、棘突间隙变窄、项韧带钝厚等。

（2）颈椎 X 线检查：正位片可见钩椎关节增生；侧位片可见颈椎生理曲度变直，椎体前缘或后缘骨质增生，椎间隙变窄，项韧带钙化。

4. Cervical Spondylosis of Sympathetic Type

（1）Muscle spasms of the neck, movement disturbance, tenderness beside the spinous process, deflection of the spinous process and parapophysis, the narrowing of interspinal interstice, and nuchal ligament hypertrophy, etc.

（2）X-ray examination of the cervical spine: The hyperplasia of luschka joint can be found in the anteroposterior film; there are straightened cervical physiological curvature, the hyperosteogeny of the anterior or posterior vertebrae, narrowing of intervertebral space, and nuchal ligament calcification in the lateral film.

5. 脊髓型颈椎病

（1）肌张力增高，肌力减退，腱反射（肱二头肌、肱三头肌、跟腱、膝腱反射）亢进，浅反射（腹壁、提睾反射）减弱或消失。

（2）病理反射（霍夫曼征、巴宾斯基征等）阳性。

（3）颈椎 MRI 检查可清楚看到椎间盘髓核及增生骨赘、黄韧带突入椎管内，压迫硬膜囊及脊髓。

5. Cervical Spondylotic Myelopathy

（1）Muscular hypertonia, reduced myodynamia, tendon hyperreflexia（biceps brachii, triceps brachii, achilles tendon, knee-jerk）; superficial reflexes（abdominal, cremasteric）are weakening or disappearing.

（2）Pathological reflexes（Hoffmann's sign, Babinski sign, etc.）show positive.

（3）Cervical spine MRI clearly shows the nucleus pulposus and hypertrophic osteophytes, that ligamentum flavum break into the spinal canal, oppressing the dural sac and spinal cord.

五、推拿治疗

治则：舒筋活血，解痉止痛，理筋整复。

Ⅴ. Tuina Treatment

Therapeutic principles: Relax muscle and accelerate circulation of blood, relieve spasm and pain, and regulate the tendon.

1. 部位及取穴

枕后部、颈肩背部、肩胛骨内缘，风池、风府、颈夹脊、大椎、肩井、天宗、阿是等穴。

1. The Location and Acupoints

The occiput posterior, neck, shoulder, back, inner edge of the scapula, Fengchi（GB 20）, Fengfu（GV16）, neck Jiaji, Dazhui（GV14）, Jianjing（GB 21）, Tianzong（SI 11）, Ashi acupoints, etc.

2. 手法

㨰、一指禅推、拿、揉、按、拔伸、扳等法。

2. Manipulation

Rolling manipulation, Yi zhi chan pushing, grasping, kneading, holding, pulling manipulations, etc.

3. 基本操作

（1）患者坐位，医生站其身后，以㨰法和一指禅推法作用于患者颈部、肩部、上背部肌肉，约 5 分钟；随后，医生一手扶病人前额部，一手拿揉颈项部，重点拿揉肌肉痉挛处，并可配合颈项部屈伸运动，反复 3—5 遍。

（2）患者坐位，医生站其身后，用拇指按揉法作用于颈部、肩背部及肩胛骨内缘痛点，反复 3—5 遍；再用拇指按风池、风府、颈夹脊、大椎、肩井、天宗、阿是等穴，每穴 1 分钟。

（3）患者坐位，医生站其身后，对棘突偏歪者进行颈椎旋转扳法，对椎动脉型及脊髓型颈椎病患者慎用或禁用扳法。

3. Basic Operations

(1) The patient is seated, while the doctor stands behind him/her using rolling manipulation and Yi zhi chan pushing manipulation with neck, shoulder, upper back muscles for about 5 minutes; Subsequently, the doctor uses one hand to hold the patient's forehead and the other hand to knead, focusing on muscle spasms, combined with flexion and extension movements of the neck. Repeat the process for 3 – 5 times.

(2) The patient is seated while the doctor stands behind him/her using the thumb-kneading manipulation with pain points in the neck, shoulder and back, and inner edge of the shoulder blade. Repeat for 3 – 5 times; then the doctor use the thumb to press Fengchi (GB 20), Fengfu (GV 16), neck Jiaji, Dazhui (GV 14), Jianjing (GB 21), Tianzong (SI 11), Ashi acupoints, 1 minute per point.

(3) The patient is seated, while the doctor stands behind him/her practicing the rotating-pulling manipulation for those with deviated spinous process to skew cervical spinous process. But the method is forbidden for the patient with cervical spondylosis of vertebral artery type and cervical spondylotic myelopathy.

4. 辩证加减

(1) 颈型颈椎病：①患者坐位，医者站其身后，对有颈椎棘突偏歪者，可施以颈椎旋转扳法，纠正偏歪棘突和关节紊乱。②患者坐位，医者站其身后，对伴有头痛者，重点用拇指按法施治于风府、风池、太阳、百会等穴；用五指拿法拿头部五经，反复3—5遍。

(2) 神经根型颈椎病：①患者坐位，医生站于一侧，对上肢有放射性疼痛和麻木者，以滚法和一指禅推法作用于患侧上肢相应神经根节段上下往返施术3—5遍。②患者坐位，医生站于一侧，以拇指按揉法作用于天鼎、肩中俞、缺盆、天宗、极泉、曲池、手三里、小海、外关、合谷、后溪等穴，每穴半分钟，按揉患侧上肢缺盆、极泉穴时，患侧上肢应有放射麻木感；再搓抖上肢，拔伸手指关节。

(3) 椎动脉型颈椎病：①患者仰卧位，医生坐其头侧，以抹法作用于印堂穴至前发际；分抹鱼腰至太阳穴，反复3—5遍。②患者仰卧位，医生坐其头侧，以指按揉法按揉睛明、印堂、百会、四神聪、太阳穴，每穴1分钟。③患者仰卧位，医生坐其头侧，以扫散法作用于头部足少阳胆经及颞部，反复3—5遍。④患者坐位，医生站其身后，以五指拿法拿头部五经，反复3—5遍。

(4) 交感神经型颈椎病：患者坐位，医生站其身后，以一指禅推法作用于风池、风府、四神聪、百会、心俞等穴，每穴1分钟。分抹桥弓，先左侧后右侧，每侧20次。

(5) 脊髓型颈椎病：①患者俯卧位，医生站于一侧，以搂、按、揉、拿等法作用于下肢部位，反复3—5遍。②患者俯卧位，医生站于一侧，以按揉法作用于环跳、秩边、承扶、阳陵泉、委中、承山、梁丘、足三里、三阴交、昆仑、太溪、涌泉等穴，每穴1分钟，以酸胀感为度。

4. Modification Based on Pattern Identification

(1) Neck type of the cervical spondylosis: ① The patient is seated while the doctor stands behind him/her, using the rotating-pulling manipulation for those with

deviated spinous process to correct the deviated spinous process and joint disorders. ② The patient is seated while the doctor stands behind him/her generally using the thumb to press Fengfu (GV 16), Fengchi (GB 20), Taiyang (EX-HN5), Baihui (GV 20) and using the fingers-grasping manipulation with the five head meridians for the patient accompanied by the headache. Repeat 3 - 5 times.

(2) Nerve root type of cervical spondylosis: ① The patient is seated while the doctor stands on one side of the patient, using the rolling manipulation and Yi zhi chan pushing manipulation in the corresponding nerve root segments of the affected upper limbs from top to bottom for those with radiating pain and numbness of the upper limb. Repeat 3 - 5 times. ② The patient is seated while the doctor stands on one side of the patient, using the thumb to press-knead Tianding (LI 17), Jian Zhongshu (LI 15), Quepen (ST 12), Tianzong (SI 11), Jiquan (HI 1), Quchi (LI 11), Shou Sanli (LI 10), Xiaohai (SI 8), Waiguan (SJ 5), Hegu (LI 4), Houxi (SI 3) and other acupoints. Each acupoint requires half of one minute. When being pressed and kneaded Quepen (ST 12) and Jiquan (HI 1) of the affected upper limb, the patient should feel radiating numbness in the affected upper limb; then the doctor rubs and shakes the upper limb and pulls the hand knuckles.

(3) Vertebral artery type of cervical spondylosis: ① The patient is lying on the back while, the doctor sits at the patient's cephalic side, using the wiping manipulation with the area from Yintang (EX-HN 3) to the anterior hairline and with the area from Yuyao (EX-HN4) to Taiyang (EX-HN5). Repeat 3 - 5 times. ② The patient is lying on the back while the doctor sits at the patient's cephalic side using the finger pressing-kneading manipulation to press and knead Jingming (BL1), Yintang (EX-HN 3), Baihui (GV 20), Si Shencong (EX-HN1), Taiyang (EX-HN5). One minute per acupoint. ③ The patient is lying on the back while the doctor sits at the patient's cephalic side, using the method of sweeping out with the gall bladder meridian in the head and tempora. Repeat 3 - 5 times. ④ The patient is seated while the doctor sits at the patient's cephalic side, using the fingers-grasping manipulation with the five head meridians. Repeat 3 - 5 times.

(4) Sympathetic type of cervical spondylosis: The patient is seated while the doctor stands behind him/her, using Yi zhi chan pushing manipulation with Fengchi (GB 20), Fengfu (GV 16), Si Shencong (EX-HN1), Baihui (GV 20), Xinshu (BL 15) and others. One minute per acupoint. Wiping Qiaogong acupoint, first on the left then the right side, 20 times each side.

(5) Cervical spondylotic myelopathy: ① The patient is lying prostrate while the doctor stands on his/her side, using rolling, pressing, kneading, grasping and other manipulations with the lower limbs. Repeat 3 - 5 times. ② The patient is lying

prostrate while the doctor stands on his/her side, using the pressing-kneading manipulation with Huantiao (GB 30), Zhibian (BL 54), Chengfu (BL 36), Yang Lingquan (GB 34), Weizhong (BL 40), Chengshan (BL 57), Liangqiu (ST 34), Zu Sanli (ST 36), Sanyin Jiao (SP 6), Kunlun (BL 60), Taixi (KI 3), Yongquan (KI 1) and others. One minute per acupoint until the patient feels soreness and distension.

六、功能锻炼

(1) 颈部前屈后伸法：在功能锻炼前进行深呼吸，吸气时使颈部尽量前屈下颌，接近胸骨柄上缘，然后在呼气时使颈部后伸至最大限度，反复7—8次。

(2) 颈部侧屈法：在深呼吸下进行，吸气时头向左偏，呼气时头部还原位，然后吸气时头向右偏，呼气时头部还原位，反复7—8次。

(3) 颈部伸展法：在深吸气时，使头颈尽量伸向左前方，呼气时使头颈还原，然后在深吸气时，使头颈尽量伸向右前方，呼气时头颈还原，反复7—8次。

(4) 颈部旋转法：头部先向左侧旋转，继而向右侧旋转，反复2—3次，然后使头颈先向左侧旋一次，再向右侧回旋一次。

(5) 意念牵引法：直立位，两足略宽于肩，双目平视，两手自然下垂，全身肌肉放松，排除杂念。然后两臂前伸上举，双手举过头顶呈十指互相交叉，翻掌缓缓上提，与此同时，随手臂上举，想象有一带子向上提拔头颈部，在意念中自觉颈部向上伸展、拉长，反复20次。

Ⅵ. Functional Exercises

(1) Neck anteflexion and posterior-extension method: take a deep breath before doing functional exercises. Bend the neck forward as much as possible when breathing in and extend the neck backward as much as possible when breathing out. Repeat 7 - 8 times.

(2) Neck lateral bending method: doing it during deep breath. Turn the head to left when breathing in and turn back when breathing out. Then turn the head right when breathing in and turn back when breathing out. Repeat 7 - 8 times.

(3) Neck stretching method: The head and neck reach out in the left-front direction as much possible when breathing deep in and turn back when breathing out. Then the head and neck reach out to the right front direction as much possible when breathing deep in and turn back when breathing out. Repeat 7 - 8 times.

(4) Neck rotation method: first, rotate the head to the left and to the right. Repeat 2 to 3 times. Then rotate the head and neck to the left for one time and to the right for one time.

(5) Mind-traction method: Stand upright with the space between the two feet slightly wider than the shoulder length, look at the front horizontally, drop the hands

naturally, relax all muscles, clear the mind. Then put the arms forward and up, put the hands above the head with the fingers crossed, turn the palms slowly and lift them. At the same time, imagine there is a belt pulling up the head and neck and that the neck extends in mind when putting the arms up. Repeat 20 times.

七、注意事项

（1）推拿手法操作宜轻巧适度，切忌暴力，以免发生意外。

（2）疼痛较甚、颈项不敢转动或脊髓型颈椎病，应选用颈围制动或卧床休息。

（3）平时加强颈部的功能锻炼，纠正日常生活中的不良习惯姿势。

（4）注意睡眠姿势，选用高低合适的枕头。避免长期低头伏案工作，注意颈肩部的保暖。

VII. Notes

（1）The manipulation should be light and moderate; do not be violent in case of accidents.

（2）Patients should have neck circumference brake or rest in bed when they feel too pain to move the neck or have cervical spondylotic myelopathy.

（3）Reinforce daily functional exercises of the neck and correct habitual bad postures in daily life.

（4）Pay attention to sleeping postures and choose a pillow that is not too high or too low. Avoid bending over one's work at desk for a long time. Keep the neck and shoulder warm.

第二节　肩关节周围炎
Section Two　Scapulohumeral Periarthritis

一、概念

肩关节周围炎是指肩关节囊和关节周围软组织损伤、退变而引起的一种慢性无菌性炎症，以肩关节疼痛、活动功能障碍和肌肉萎缩为临床主要特征的疾病，简称肩周炎，又称为"五十肩""冻结肩""肩凝症""漏肩风"等。

本病以体力劳动者为多见，女性略多于男性，且常发生在单侧肩部，多见于 50 岁左右的女性。本病属中医"肩痹"范畴。

I. Definition

Scapulohumeral periarthritis is a chronic aseptic inflammation caused by injury and degeneration of capsula articularis humeri and articular peripheral soft tissues. The main clinical symptoms include shoulder pain, activity dysfunction and muscle atrophy. The disease is also known as "fifty shoulder" "frozen shoulder" "inability to raise shoulder" or "Lou Jian Feng (leak shoulder wind)".

The disease is more common in manual workers and around 50-year-old women, often occurring in the unilateral shoulder. The disease is categorized under "shoulder Bi (impediment)" in traditional Chinese medicine.

二、病因病理

肩关节是人体活动范围最广泛的关节，其关节囊较松弛。维持肩关节的稳定性，多数依靠其周围的肌肉、肌腱和韧带的力量。跨越肩关节的肌腱、韧带较多，而且大多是细长的肌腱，由于肌腱本身的血供较差，随着年龄的增长，常有退行性改变；另一方面由于肩关节在日常生活和劳动中活动比较频繁。双肩部软组织经常受到上肢重力和肩关节大范围运动的牵拉、扭转，容易引起损伤和劳损。损伤后，软组织的充血、水肿、渗出、增厚等炎性改变如得不到有效的治疗，久之则可发生肩关节软组织粘连形成，甚至肌腱钙化，导致肩关节活动功能严重障碍。

Ⅱ. Etiology and Pathology

Shoulder joint is the most extensive one in human body activities, but its capsula articularis humeri is looser than any other. The stability of shoulder joint mostly relies on the strength of muscle, tendon and ligament around. There are more tendon and ligament across shoulder joint, most of which are slender. For the poor blood supply, tendon tends to have degenerative changes with age. In another way, shoulder joint activity is more frequent in daily life and labor. Shoulder soft tissues are often damaged by the pulling and twisting due to upper limbs gravity and the large overall motion of shoulder joint. After damage, congestion, edema, exudation, thickening and other inflammatory changes of the soft tissues, if not given effective treatment tend to develop into shoulder joint soft tissue desmoplasia or tendon calcification, resulting in serious shoulder joint activity dysfunction.

三、临床表现

1. 肩部疼痛

初期常感肩部前上方、肱二头肌短头附着点、结节间沟及肩峰下方的三角肌附着点多处疼痛，疼痛可急性发作，多数呈慢性。常因天气变化和劳累后诱发。初期疼痛为阵发性，后期逐渐发展成持续性酸痛，并逐渐加重，昼轻夜重，夜不能寐。肩部受牵拉或碰撞后，可引起剧烈疼痛。肩部怕风、怕冷，不敢向患侧卧。疼痛可持续几个月至一年不等。

2. 功能障碍

早期功能障碍多因疼痛所致,后期疼痛减轻而肩关节广泛粘连,致肩关节各方向活动功能受限,尤以外展、内收、内旋及后伸功能受限为甚。特别是当肩关节外展时,出现典型的"扛肩"现象。梳头、穿衣等动作均难以完成。日久,则可发生三角肌等失用性萎缩。

Ⅲ. Clinical Manifestations

1. Shoulder Pain

In the early stage of the disease, the patient often feels pain on the multiple places, such as the anterior shoulder, attachment points of coracoradialis, intertubercular sulcus, attachment points of deltoid below acromion. The pains are acute, but mostly chronic. It can be induced by weather changes and tiredness. In the early time of disease, the pain start as paroxysmal pain, but in the later time, it gradually develops into persistent pain. The pain relieves in the day, but at night it aggravates even to an extent that the patient can't sleep well. Crashed or stretched shoulder can lead to intense pains. With shoulder aversion of cold and wind, the patient can't bear to sleep on affected side. The pain can last several mouths even one year or two.

2. Dysfunction

In the early time of disease, the dysfunction is mostly caused by pain, but in later time, pain relieves but shoulder joint adhesion occurs, giving rise to the impaired functions of shoulder motions, especially the motion of abduction, adduction, intorsion and backward extension. When shoulder joint abducts, the typical symptom of elevated shoulder will present, which makes actions like combing hair or dressing different to complete. In a long term, the deltoid and other muscles may atrophy due to disuse.

四、诊断要点

(1)肩部有外伤、劳损或感受风寒湿邪的病史。

(2)肩部疼痛,疼痛的性质多为钝痛,活动时疼痛加剧,且可向上臂及肘部放射。

(3)压痛较广泛,常见于喙突、肩峰下、三角肌附着处结节间沟、肩后部、肩胛骨内侧缘等。

(4)肩关节活动受限。

(5)肩部肌肉萎缩。

(6)X线检查:一般无异常,后期可出现骨质疏松、关节间隙变窄或增宽以及骨质增生、软组织钙化等。肩关节造影可见关节囊有粘连现象。

Ⅳ. Diagnostic Points

（1）The patient has a medical history of shoulder trauma, shoulder strain or contractions of wind-cold-dampness evil.

（2）Shoulder pain, mostly dull pain, worsens during movement and radiates to upper arm and elbow.

（3）Extensive tenderness in coracoid, subacromial, intertubercular sulcus of the attachment of deltoid muscle, the back shoulder and the internal edge of scapula.

（4）Shoulder activities is limited.

（5）Shoulder muscles atrophy.

（6）X-ray examination: Generally no abnormalities are present. But in later stage, the abnormalities like osteoporosis, narrowed or widened joint space, hyperostosis, and calcified soft tissue will occur. With shoulder joint contrast, articular capsule adhesion can be seen.

五、推拿治疗

治则：温通经络,活血止痛,松解粘连,滑利关节。

1. 部位及穴位

肩臂部,肩井、肩髃、肩内陵、秉风、天宗、肩贞、曲池、手三里、合谷等穴。

2. 手法

揉、拿、点、弹拨、摇、扳、搓、抖等法。

3. 操作

（1）患者坐位,医生站于患侧,以一手托住患者上臂使其微外展,另一手施滚法或拿揉法于肩臂部,约 3 分钟,重点在肩前部、三角肌部及肩后部,同时配合患肢的被动外展、旋外和旋内活动,以温通经络。

（2）患者坐位,医生站于患侧,以点压、弹拨法依次点压、弹拨肩井、秉风、天宗、肩内陵、肩贞、肩髃等穴,约 5 分钟,以酸胀为度。

（3）患者坐位,医生站于患侧,对有粘连部位或痛点施弹拨法,以解痉止痛、剥离粘连。

（4）患者坐位,医生站于患侧,一手扶住患肩,另一手握住其腕部或托住肘部,以肩关节为轴心作环转摇动,幅度由小到大,反复 10 次;然后作肩关节内收、外展、后伸及内旋的扳动各 5 次。医生施拿捏法于肩部周围,约 2 分钟,然后握住患者腕部,将患肢慢慢提起,使其上举,并同时作牵拉提抖,反复 10 次。

（5）患者坐位,医生站于患侧,以搓法从肩部到前臂,反复上下搓动 3—5 遍,并牵抖患肢 1 分钟。

Ⅴ. Tuina Treatment

Principle of Treatment: promoting the flow of qi by warming the channel, promoting blood circulation and relieving pain, removing adhesion and lubricating joint.

1. Locations and Acupoints

The region of shoulder and arm, Jianjing (GB 21), Jianyu (LI 15), Jian Neiling (EX-UE12), Bingfeng (SI 12), Tianzong (SI 11), Jianzhen (SI 19), Quchi (LI 11), Shou Sanli (LI 10), Hegu (LI 4), etc.

2. Manipulation

Rolling, kneading, grasping, pointing, flicking and poking, rotating, pulling, foulage, shaking, etc.

3. Operation

(1) The patient is in a sitting position, the doctor stands by the patient's affected side, with his hand holding the patient's arm to make it abduct and the other hand keeping rolling, taking up and rubbing the should and arm, especially the anterior shoulder, deltoid muscle and posterior shoulder, for about 3 minutes. And the whole process should be accompanied with the passive movement of the affected joint like abduction, lateral rotation and medial rotation in order to promote qi and warm the channel.

(2) The patient is seated, while the doctor stands on the patient's affected side, pointing, flicking and poking the points Jianjing (GB 21), Bingfeng (SI 12), Tianzong (SI 11), Jian Neiling (EX-UE12), Jianzhen (SI 19), Jianyu (LI 15) in turn for about 5 minutes until the patient feels sore and swelling.

(3) The patient is in a sitting position, while the doctor stands by the patient's affected side, relieving spasm and pain and striping adhesion by flicking and poking the adhesive region or aching point.

(4) The patient is in a sitting position. The doctor stands by the patient's affected side, with one hand supporting the patient's shoulder and the other holding the patient on the wrist and elbow, and keeps moving the arm around the axis of the shoulder joint for 10 times. Then the doctor pulls the shoulder joint in the direction of adduction, abduction, extension and intorsion for five times, respectively. After pulling, grasp and pinch the shoulder for 2 minutes and then hold the wrist of the affected arm and elevate it. At the same time, shake it and then pull it for 10 times.

(5) The patient is in a sitting position, while the doctor stands by the patient's affected side, twisting the affected arm up and down for 3 - 5 times and shaking it for a minute.

六、功能锻炼

1. 壁虎爬墙法

患者面对墙壁用双手或患侧单手沿墙壁缓慢向上摸高爬动，使患肢尽量上举，然后再缓慢向下回到原处，反复进行，循序渐进，不断提高爬墙高度，也可让患者站在单杠下用单手或双手握住单杠对肩关节进行牵拉，以解除粘连。

2. 臂环转运动法

患者站立，单臂或双臂由前向后数次，再由后向前数次，做环转活动。

3. 上肢背伸法

双手向后背伸，用健手拉住患肢腕部，逐渐向上提拉，反复进行。

4. 外旋运动法

背部紧靠墙壁而立，上臂紧贴身体两侧，屈肘90°握拳，做肩关节外旋动作，幅度逐渐增大至最大活动范围，反复进行。

Ⅵ. Functional Exercises

1. Climbing the Wall like a Wall Lizard

The patient should face the wall with his two hands or only the affected one climbing up the walls slowly to raise the arm(s) to the greatest extent. Then replace the hands (hand) slowly. Repeat the movement for several times and increase the height step by step. The patient can also hold the horizontal bar by one or both hands and tract to remove adhesion.

2. Rotating the Arm(s)

The patient is in a standing position with his arm or both arms protruding from front to back for several times and another several times in reverse to rotate the arm(s).

3. Stretching the Arms to the Back

Stretch the arms to the back and the healthy hand holds the wrist of the affected upper limb and raise it gradually. Repeat the exercises.

4. Lateral Rotating Exercises

Stand against the wall with the arms close to the body and the elbow bent 90°. Clench the fist and rotate the shoulder joint laterally. Increase the range gradually till to the greatest extent and repeat.

七、注意事项

运用手法要轻柔，不可施用猛力，以免造成骨折或脱位等严重损伤。注意局部保暖，防止受凉，以免加重病情，影响治疗效果。进行适当的肩部功能锻炼，并遵循持之以恒，循序渐进。

Ⅶ. Notes

The manipulation should be gentle rather than vigorous to avoid severe injury like fracture and dislocation. Keep local warm and prevent cold to avoid aggravating the illness and impacting the effects. Keep proper functional shoulder exercises and follow it step by step.

第三节　腰椎间盘突出症
Section Three　Lumbar Disc Herniation

一、概念

腰椎间盘突出症是指由于腰椎间盘变性、纤维环破裂,髓核突出刺激或压迫神经根、马尾神经所引起的以腰痛并伴有一侧或双侧下肢放射性疼痛等症状为特征的一种综合征,简称"腰突症",又称为"腰椎间盘纤维环破裂症"。

本病临床十分常见,好发于青壮年,男性多于女性,且以 20—40 岁居多。由于下腰部负重大、活动多,腰椎间盘突出症多发于第 4—5 腰椎及第 5 腰椎与第 1 骶椎之间的椎间盘。本病属中医"痹症""腰痛"范畴。

Ⅰ. Definition

Lumbar disc herniation is a kind of syndrome caused by degeneration of the lumbar intervertebral disc, tear of the fibrous ring, herniation of the nucleus pulposus, compression of the nerve root or the cauda equina. It is characterized with lumbago and pain radiating to one side or two sides of lower limb. Thus, it is called lumbar protrusion for short and also called "tear of lumbar intervertebral disc's fibrous ring".

Commonly seen in clinical, it is vulnerable to the young, especially those between the age of 20 to 40. Male is more frequently affected than female. Because the heavy weight-bearing and over activity of the low waist, the lumbar intervertebral disc protrusion most attack the intervertebral disc between the 4th and 5th lumbar vertebra and between the 5th lumbar vertebra and the first sacral vertebra. This disease belongs to Bi Syndrome or lumbago in TCM.

二、病因病理

1. 内因

（1）解剖结构:腰椎间盘纤维环后外侧较为薄弱,加之后纵韧带自第一腰椎平面以下逐渐变窄,至第五腰椎和第一骶椎间后纵韧带只有原来的一半。而腰骶部是承受动、静力最大的部位,故后纵韧带的变窄,造成了自然结构的弱点,使髓核易向后方两侧突出。

(2)椎间盘退变:人体青春期后,各种组织即出现退行性变化,其中椎间盘的退变发生较早,主要是髓核脱水,椎间盘失去其正常的弹性和张力,在此基础上由于较重的外伤或多次反复不明显的损伤,造成纤维环软弱或破裂,髓核即由该处突出,从一侧(少数可同时在两侧)的侧后方突入椎管,也可由中央向后突出。

2. 外因

由于外力作用或风寒之邪刺激,导致腰脊柱内外力失衡,突出的髓核刺激周围组织产生损伤性炎症变化,形成混合性突出物,刺激或压迫神经根而产生神经根受损伤征象;压迫马尾神经,造成大小便障碍;进入椎管,可造成广泛的马尾神经损害。

Ⅱ. Etiology and Pathology

1. Intrinsic Factor

(1) Anatomical structure: The posterior and lateral fibrous ring of lumbar intervertebral disc is thin, and the posterior longitudinal ligament becomes narrow down from the plane of the first lumbar vertebra and remains half on the plane between the 5th lumbar vertebra and the first sacral vertebra. Lumbosacral portion bears the heaviest dynamic strength and static force, so the narrowed posterior longitudinal ligament is the weakness which makes the nucleus pulposus herniate to the back from two sides easily.

(2) Degeneration of the intervertebral disc: After puberty, the tissues in human body begin to degenerate. The degeneration of the intervertebral disc appears earlier. The most obvious variation is water deprivation of nucleus pulposus, making the intervertebral disc lose its flexibility and tension. On this basis, with severe trauma or repeated invisible injury, the fibrous ring becomes weak or even ruptures, and the nucleus pulposus will herniate from one side or both two sides to spinal canal, or it can also herniate to the back from the center.

2. External Factor

Exogenic action or cold attack leads to the unbalance between the internal and external force of vertebral column. The protruded nucleus pulposus stimulates the tissues around, causing traumatic inflammation and forming mixed outshoot. The mixed prominence stimulates or compresses the nerve root, impairing the nerve root. It can also compress the cauda equina nerve, resulting in the disorders of urination and defecation. Or if it enters into the spinal canal, it will damage the cauda equina nerve extensively.

三、临床表现

腰部疼痛,可持续疼痛,也可反复发作,严重者不能久坐、久立、久行,翻身转侧困难,休息后症状减轻。下肢放射性疼痛,可与腰痛同时出现,也可单独出现,咳嗽、大便用力、打喷嚏时疼痛及放射性疼痛加重。腰部前屈、后伸、侧弯、旋转等活动受限。久病患者,常有主观麻木感,多局限于小腿后外侧、足背、足跟或足掌。中央型髓核突出可发生鞍区麻痹,甚至膀胱、直肠功能障碍。患侧下肢有发凉感。

Ⅲ. Clinical Manifestations

Waist pain that can be continuous or repetitive. Patients with severe lumbar intervertebral disc protrusion couldn't sit, stand or walk for a long time, or couldn't turn over easily. The symptom can relieve after a rest. Pain radiating to the lower limbs may appear alone or along with the waist pain. The pain or the radiating pain worsens when the patient is coughing, defecating hard or sneezing. Activities like bending forward, backward, laterally or rotating are limited. Person who falling ill for a long time would often feel numb in the posterolateral shank, acrotarsium, heel and sole. Central herniation of the nucleus pulposus can cause paralysis of sellar region, even dysfunction of bladder or rectum. Patient would feel cool in the lower limbs.

四、诊断要点

(1) 腰痛伴下肢放射性疼痛、麻木。腹压增高时,则腰腿痛加剧。

(2) 腰4—5或腰5骶1棘间韧带侧方可触及明显的压痛点,按压痛点时,可引起小腿或足部的放射性疼痛;多数患者有不同程度的腰脊柱侧弯,生理前凸减小或消失,甚至后弓;腰活动受限。

(3) 屈颈试验阳性,严重者坐位屈颈试验不能完成;挺腹试验阳性;直腿抬高试验及加强试验阳性。

(4) 小腿前外或后外侧皮肤感觉减退,患侧跟腱反射减退或消失,甚至肌肉萎缩。根据突出椎间盘位置的不同,可以出现足背伸跖屈肌力的减弱。

(5) X线检查:可见脊柱侧弯、椎间隙变窄、椎体边缘唇状增生。

(6) CT、MRI检查:可见椎间盘后缘或后侧缘有局限性软组织密度影突向椎管,有时突出物伴有钙化,同时可见黄韧带增厚、侧隐窝狭窄等;椎管与硬膜囊之间的脂肪层消失;或可见硬膜囊受压移位和神经根受压移位;有时可见突出物突破后纵韧带而游离于硬膜外间隙中。

Ⅳ. Diagnostic Points

(1) Lumbago with pain radiating to the lower limbs, numbness. The pain will aggravate when the abdominal pressure rises.

(2) Obvious tenderness can be touched on the $L_4 \sim L_5$ or the side of the interspinous ligament of L_5 and S_1. When pressing the pain points, the pain will radiate to the lower leg or the foot. Most patients have waist lateral curvature in various degrees, decreased or disappeared lordosis, even posterior curvature, and limited waist activity.

(3) Linder's sign is positive. If it is severe, the patient can't do this test while seated. Very belly test is positive. Straighten belly test, the straight leg raise test and the intensified one are all positive.

(4) Reduced sensation on the antero-lateral or posterior-lateral legs, reduced or disappeared reflection of the achilles's tendon on the affected side, atrophied muscles. The force of dorsiflexion plantar flexor may reduce depending on the different locations of herniated disc.

(5) X-ray examination: Lateral curvature, narrowed intervertebral space, liplike hyperplasia on the edge of vertebral are seen in the X-ray examination.

(6) CT, MRI examination: CT and MRI examination may show limited soft tissue density protruding towards the vertebral canal in the posterior or posterolateral intervertebral disc. Sometimes the calcified protrusion, thickened ligamentum flava, narrowed lateral crypt are accompanied. The adipose layer between vertebral canal and dural sac is disappeared. The dural sac and the nerve root are pressed and displaced. Sometimes the protrusion will break out of the posterior longitudinal ligament and wandered in the epidural space.

五、推拿治疗

治则：疏经通络，解痉止痛，行气活血，理筋整复。

1. 部位及取穴

背腰部、下肢部，肾俞、大肠俞、腰阳关、环跳、承扶、殷门、委中、承山、昆仑等穴。

2. 手法

㨰、按、揉、拔伸、弹拨、扳、擦、运动关节等法。

3. 操作

(1) 患者俯卧位，医生站于一侧，先以滚法在脊柱两侧膀胱经施术 3—5 分钟，以腰部为重点；然后再以㨰法在患侧臀部及下肢后外侧部施术，3—5 分钟。

(2) 患者俯卧位，医生站于一侧，分别以按揉、弹拨等法在患侧腰臀部及下肢后外侧施术 5—7 分钟,以改善肌肉紧张痉挛状态。

(3)患者俯卧位,医生站于一侧,以拇指或肘尖点压腰阳关、肾俞、居髎、环跳、承扶、委中、阿是等穴;横擦腰骶部,以透热为度。

(4)患者俯卧位,医生站于一侧,在助手配合拔伸牵引的情况下,医生以拇指顶推或肘尖按压患处,使椎间隙增宽,增加盘外压力,降低盘内压力,促使突出的髓核回纳,减轻突出物对神经根的压迫,并且增强腰部肌肉组织的痛阈。

(5)患者侧卧位,医生站于一侧,以腰部斜扳法,左右各一次,以调整后关节紊乱,松解粘连,改变突出物与神经根的位置。然后再嘱患者仰卧位,强制直腿抬高以牵拉坐骨神经与腘绳肌,可起到松解粘连的作用,并可使脊椎后部和后纵韧带牵拉,增加椎间盘外周的压力,相对减轻了盘内的压力,从而迫使髓核变位或复位。

Ⅴ. Tuina Treatment

Principle of Treatment: Dredging the meridians, relieving spasm and pain, promoting the circulation of qi and blood, restoring injured muscular tendon.

1. Position and Acupoint Selection

Back and waist, lower limbs, Shenshu (BL 23), Dachang shu (BL 25), Yao yangguan (GV 3), Huantiao (GB 30), Chengfu (BL 36), Yinmen (BL 37), Weizhong (BL 40), Chengshan (BL 57), Kunlun (BL 60), ect.

2. Technique

Rolling, pressing, kneading, drawing, plucking, pulling, rubbing, moving joints, ect.

3. Operation

(1) The patient is in prone position, while the doctor stands beside the patient. Apply the rolling manipulation first on bladder meridians beside the backbone for 3 - 5 minutes, with the focus on the waist, and then roll the buttock and the lateral and posterior lower limb of the affected side for about 3 - 5 minutes.

(2) With the patient in prone position, the doctor stands beside the patient and massages the patients' wrist and the posterolateral lower limbs by pressing, kneading and flicking for about 5～7 minutes so as to relieve muscle spasm.

(3) With the patient in prone position, the doctor stands beside the patient and presses the patients' acupoints such as Yao yangguan (GV 3), Shenshu (BL 23), Juliao (GB 29), Huantiao (GB 30), Chengfu (BL 36), Weizhong (BL 40), Ashi acupoint and so on with thumb or elbow; rub the wrist to warm the body.

(4) With the patient in prone position, the doctor stands beside the patient. With the assistant pulling and stretching the patient, the doctor pushes upward the affected area with the thumb or presses the affected part with elbow point to enlarge the space

between the vertebrae, to increase the pressure inside intervertebral discs and to decrease the pressure outside. In this way, the protruding nucleus pulposus can be reset to relieve the pressure of nerve root and to raise the pain threshold of waist muscles and tissues.

(5) The patient lies on one side, while the doctor stands by one side and pulls the wrist once on both sides to adjust the disorder of joint, release the adhesion tendon and change the position of the protruded disc and the nerve root. Then let the patient lie on his back and force him to do straight-leg raising exercise so as to strength sciatic nerve and hamstring tendon to relieve the adhesion. At the same time, stretch the back of the spine and posterior longitudinal ligament to increase the pressure inside intervertebral discs and decrease the pressure outside to adjust the nucleus pulposus.

六、功能锻炼

1. 背伸锻炼法

患者俯卧,双下肢伸直,两手放在身体两旁,两腿不动,抬头时上身躯体向后背伸,每日3次,每次做20—50次。经过一段时间的锻炼,适应后改为抬头后伸及双下肢直腿后伸,同时腰部尽量背伸,每日5—10次,每次做50—100次,以锻炼腰背部肌肉力量。

2. 倒走法

于地面平整、较为空旷之处,行倒走训练。倒走时,可摆动双臂以保持身体平衡。初时,须注意避免跌跤,每次约10分钟;熟练后,可酌情延长。此法可调整腰臀肌功能,贵在坚持。

Ⅵ. Functional Exercises

1. Stretching Back Method

In a prone position, the patient keeps two legs straight with both hands at his sides. Keep the legs still and the upper body stretch backwards when raising the head. It should be done three times per day and each time for 20~50 rounds. After a period of exercise, the patient can extend the head and two lower limbs backward, and stretch back as much as possible for 5 to 10 times per day to strengthen the muscles of the back.

2. Inverted Walking Method

Walk backwards in the open ground. Swinging arms is recommended to keep balance. At the beginning, watch out to avoid falling and exercise for 10 minutes every time and prolong the time later. This method can adjust the function of wrist and buttock muscle. Do it persistently.

七、注意事项

(1) 推拿治疗前应排除骨、关节疾病及推拿禁忌证。

(2) 手法操作应柔和,避免使用暴力和蛮力。

(3) 推拿治疗时,对突出物巨大或有钙化者、马尾神经受压者、继发椎管狭窄者,应慎用后伸扳法。

(4) 治疗期间,患者宜卧硬板床休息,并注意腰部保暖,尽量避免弯腰动作。

(5) 病情好转后,适当进行腰背肌肉功能锻炼,促进康复。

Ⅶ. Notes

(1) Before tuina, those with bone or joint diseases need to be excluded, so do those with contraindications of tuina.

(2) Be gentle and avoid using forceful or violent forces.

(3) Avoid using pulling method when the bulge is too large or calcified, or the cauda equine is pressed or secondary spinal stenosis is seen. .

(4) During the treatment, the patient should sleep in firm bed and keep warm. Don't bend the waist.

(5) When the patient gets better, moderate exercise of back and waist muscles is recommended to promote recovery.

第四节　头　痛
Section Four　Headache

一、概念

头痛通常是指局限于头颅上半部分,包括眉弓、耳轮上缘和枕外隆突连线以上部位的疼痛,为临床常见的症状。可单独出现,也可兼见于多种急、慢性疾病中。

西医将头痛大致分为原发性和继发性两类,前者也可称为特发性头痛,常见的如偏头痛、紧张型头痛;后者包括各种颅内病变如脑血管疾病、颅内感染、颅脑外伤,全身性疾病和滥用精神活性药物等。头痛一年四季、任何年龄均可发生。本病属中医"头风""脑风"等范畴。

Ⅰ. Definition

Headache is a kind of pain usually limited to the upper part of the head, including the area beyond the line connecting the eyebrow, upper edge of the helix and the external occipital protuberance, and it is a common clinical symptom. It can appear alone, and also can be found in a variety of acute and chronic diseases.

In western medicine, headache can be divided into two categories, primary disease and secondary disease. The former can be called idiopathic headache, such as migraine, tension headache; the latter includes various intracranial lesions such as cerebrovascular disease, intracranial infection, craniocerebral trauma, systemic disease and misuse of psychoactive drugs. Headache can occur at any age or in any season. It belongs to "head wind" or "brain wind" in traditional Chinese medicine.

二、病因病机

中医认为头痛与外感风寒及头部外伤、外感风热之邪及情志内伤和肝郁阳亢、外感暑湿之邪及中焦阻塞、血虚及肾亏有关。

西医认为头痛的发病机制复杂,主要是由于颅内、外痛敏结构内的痛觉感受器受到刺激,经痛觉传导通路传导到达大脑皮层而引起。可见于现代医学内、外、神经、五官等各科疾病中。

Ⅱ. Etiology and Pathology

Traditional Chinese medicine believes that headache is associated with the affection of wind-cold and head injury, affection of wind-heat and emotional stress, affection of dampness in the summer and blocking of middle energizer and blood-insufficiency and deficiency of the kidney.

It is considered that the mechanism of headache is complicated in western medicine. The main reason is pain receptor in intracranial and extracranial pain sensitivity structure is stimulated, and it transmits pain by pain channel to the cerebral cortex to cross pain. It can be seen in a series of diseases in internal medicine, surgical medicine, department of neurology and ophthalmology and otorhinolaryngologymodern medicine.

三、辨证分型

(1) 风寒头痛：多发于吹风受寒之后引起头痛,有时痛连项背,恶风寒,喜裹头,口不渴,苔薄白,脉浮或紧。

(2) 风热头痛：头胀痛,甚则如裂,恶风发热,面红目赤,口渴欲饮,咽红肿痛,尿黄或便秘,苔薄黄或舌尖红,脉浮数。

(3) 暑湿头痛：头痛如裹,脘闷纳呆,肢体倦怠,身热汗出,心烦口渴,苔腻,脉濡数。

(4) 肝阳头痛：头痛眩晕,心烦易怒,睡眠不安,面红口干,苔薄黄或舌红少苔,脉弦或弦细数。

(5) 痰浊头痛：头痛头胀,胸膈支满,纳呆倦怠,口吐涎沫,恶心,苔白腻,脉滑。

(6) 血虚头痛：头痛头晕,神疲乏力,面色少华,心悸气短,舌淡,脉细无力。

(7) 肾亏头痛：头脑空痛,耳鸣目眩,腰酸腿软,遗精带下;阳虚者四肢作冷,舌淡胖,脉沉细无力,阴虚者口干少津,舌质红,脉细数。

(8) 瘀血头痛：头痛时作,经久不愈,痛处固定,痛如锥刺,舌有瘀斑,脉涩。

Ⅲ. Pattern Differentiation

(1) Headache due to wind-cold: It often occurs after affection of wind-cold, sometimes together with neck or back pain, aversion to wind and cold, preference to wrap the head, not thirst, thin white fur and floating or tense pulse.

(2) Headache due to wind-heat: It is characterized with swelling pain of the head, or even splitting headache, aversion to wind, fever, brush face and red eyes, thirst with desire to drink water, a swollen throat, yellow urine and constipation, red tip of the tongue, thin yellow coating and floating and quick pulse.

(3) Headache due to summer-dampness: It is featured with head as heavy as swathed, abdominal distension, poor appetite, fatigue, feeling hot and sweating, upset and thirst, greasy fur, and slippery and quick pulse.

(4) Headache due to liver-*yang*: It is characterized with headache and dizziness, upset and irritation, unquiet sleep, thirst with brush face, thin yellow fur or red tongue with little fur, wiry pulse or wiry, thready and quick pulse.

(5) Headache due to phlegm: It is featured with swelling pain of the head, a sense of chest suppression, fatigue with a poor appetite, slobbering and nausea, white greasy coating and slippery pulse.

(6) Headache due to blood-deficiency: It is characterized with headache and dizziness, fatigue, pale complexion, palpitation and shortness of breath, pale tongue, and thready and weak pulse.

(7) Headache due to deficiency of the kidney: It is characterized with empty pain of the head, tinnitus and dizziness, soreness and weakness of waist and knees, spermatorrhea and morbid leucorrhea. If yang is deficient, there are symptoms of cold limbs, pale and corpulent tongue, collapsing and thready and weak pulse; if yin is deficient, there are symptoms of dry mouth with little fluid, red tongue, and thready and quick pulse.

(8) Headache due to blood stasis: It is featured with accidental headache that can't be cured for long time. The stabbing pain is fixed with ecchymosis on the tongue and unsmooth pulse.

四、诊断要点

(1) 以头痛为主症,其部位可在前额、额颞、巅顶、顶枕部或全头部,头痛性质多为跳痛、刺痛、胀痛、昏痛、隐痛等。

(2) 头痛有突然而作,其痛如破而无休止者;也有反复发作,久治不愈,时痛时止者;头痛每次发作可持续数分钟、数小时、数天或数周不等。

（3）因外感、内伤等因素，突然而病或有反复发作的病史。

（4）应行血常规、血压、颅脑 CT 等检查，有助于排除器质性疾病。

Ⅳ. Diagnostic Points

（1）Headache is the main symptom. The position can be found on the forehead, or frontal and temporal part, or parietal part, or parietal and occipital part, or whole head. The pain may be jumping, stabbing, swelling and indistinct or dull.

（2）Headache may occur suddenly, and it is splitting and never stops; it may occur recurrently and can't be cured for long time, and it sometimes occurs and sometimes stops; it may last for several minutes or hours or days or weeks and etc.

（3）The factors may be external and internal, and the headache may occur suddenly or recurrently.

（4）Routine examination should include routine blood test, blood pressure examination, brain CT and etc to eliminate organic diseases.

五、推拿治疗

1. 治疗原则

舒筋通络、活血化瘀、解痉止痛。风寒头痛者辅以疏风散寒；风热头痛者辅以疏风清热；暑湿头痛者辅以祛暑胜湿；肝阳头痛者辅以平肝息风；痰浊头痛者辅以健脾化痰；血虚头痛者辅以滋阴养血；肾虚头痛者辅以补肾生髓；瘀血头痛者辅以活血化瘀。

2. 部位及穴位

项部和前额部，风池、风府、天柱、印堂、头维、太阳、鱼腰、百会等穴。

3. 手法

一指禅推、拿、按、揉等法。

4. 基本操作

患者坐位。医生以一指禅推法沿项部两侧上下往返治疗，3—5 分钟；按揉风池、风府、天柱等穴，2—3 分钟；拿两侧风池，并沿项部两侧自上而下操作 4—5 遍。一指禅推法从印堂开始，向上沿前额发际至头维，再至太阳，往返 3—5 遍。按揉印堂、鱼腰、太阳、百会等穴，2—3 分钟。五指拿法从头顶拿至风池穴，改用三指拿法，沿膀胱经拿至大椎两侧，往返 3—5 遍。

5. 辩证加减

（1）风寒头痛：按揉项背部 2—3 分钟，重点按揉肺俞、风门穴；拿肩井穴 30 次；小鱼际擦法直擦背部两侧膀胱经，以透热为度。

（2）风热头痛：按揉大椎、肺俞、风门穴，每穴 1 分钟；拿肩井穴 30 次；按法结合拿法按拿曲池、合谷穴，以酸胀为度；拍击背部两侧膀胱经，以皮肤微红为度。

（3）暑湿头痛：按揉大椎、曲池穴，每穴 1 分钟；拿肩井、合谷穴，以酸胀为度；拍击背部两侧膀胱经,以皮肤微红为度;提捏印堂及项部皮肤,以皮肤透红为度。

(4)肝阳头痛:推桥弓,自上而下,每侧各20余次,两侧交替进行;扫散法在头侧胆经循行部自前上方向后下方操作,两侧交替进行,各数十次,并配合按角孙穴;按揉太冲、行间穴,以酸胀为度;掌擦法斜擦涌泉穴,以透热为度。

(5)痰浊头痛:一指禅推中脘、天枢穴,每穴1—2分钟;摩腹3分钟;按揉脾俞、胃俞、大肠俞、足三里、丰隆、内关穴,每穴1分钟;掌擦法横擦左侧背部,以透热为度。

(6)血虚头痛:摩腹5分钟,以中脘、气海、关元穴为重点;掌擦法直擦背部督脉,以透热为度;按揉心俞、膈俞、足三里、三阴交穴,以微微酸胀为度。

(7)肾虚头痛:摩腹5分钟,以气海、关元穴为重点;掌擦法直擦背部督脉,横擦腰部肾俞、命门穴及腰骶部,均以透热为度。

(8)瘀血头痛:按揉太阳、攒竹穴,每穴1分钟;分抹前额和头侧胆经循行部位3—5遍;掌擦前额及两侧太阳穴部位,以透热为度。

Ⅴ. Tuina Treatment

1. Principles

Relax tendons and unlock the channels, activate blood circulation and dissipate blood stasis, relieve spasm and pain. For headache due to wind-cold, expel wind and cold pathogens; for headache due to wind-heat, dissipate wind and heat pathogens; for headache due to summer-dampness, eliminate summer-heat and remove dampness; for headache due to hyperactivity of liver-yang, calm liver-wind; for headache due to phlegm, strengthen the spleen and reduce phlegm: for headache due to blood-deficiency, enrich yin-fluid and nourish the blood; for headache due to deficiency of the kidney, tonify the kidney; for headache due to blood stasis, activate blood circulation and dissipate blood stasis.

2. Position and Acupoint

Nape and forehead, Fengchi (GB 20), Fengfu (GV 16), Tianchu (BL 10), Yintang (EX-HN 3), Touwei(ST 8), Taiyang (EX-HN5), Yuyao (EX-HN4), Baihui (GV 20) and etc.

3. Manipulation

YI zhi chan pushing, grasping, pressing, kneading manipulation etc.

4. Basic Manipulations

The doctor pushes along the two sides of the napex by Yi zhi chan pushing for about three to five minutes. Press and knead acupoints of Fengchi (GB 20), Fengfu (GV 16), Tianchu (BL 10) for two to three minutes. Grasp Fengchi (GB 20) acupoints from up to down for four to five times. Push from Yintang (EX-HN 3) to the hairline of the forehead and Touwei (ST 8) and then Taiyang (EX-HN5) for three to five times back and forth. Press and knead acupoints of Yintang（EX-HN 3），Yuyao（EX-HN4），Taiyang（EX-HN5），Baihui（GV20）for about two to three minutes. Grasp with five fingers from the top of the head to Fengchi（GB 20），then grasp with there fingers the two sides of Dazhui（GV 14）along urinary bladder meridian for three to five times back and forth.

5. Dialectical Addition and Subtraction

（1）Headache due to wind-cold: Press and knead napex and back for two to three minutes, particularly press and knead acupoints of Feishu（BL 13），Fengmen（BL 12）；grasp Jianjing（GB 21）for thirsty times; rub directly along the two sides of bladder meridian of the back by your hypothenar eminence, till the skin becomes warmer.

（2）Headache due to wind-heat: Press and knead Dazhui（GV 14），Feishu（BL 13），Fengmen（BL 12），each point for one minute; grasp Jianjing（GB 21）for thirsty times; press and grasp acupoints of Quchi（LI 11），Hegu（LI 4）with the association of pressing and grasping manipulations, till the patient feels sour; clap two sides of bladder meridian of the back, till the skin turns into red slightly.

（3）Headache due to summer-dampness: Press and knead Dazhui（GV 14）and Quchi（LI 11），each point for one minute; grasp Jianjing（GB 21）and Hegu（LI 4）till the patient feels sour; clap the two sides of bladder meridian of the back till the skin turns into slightly red; pinch the skin around Yintang（EX-HN 3）and the napex till the skin turns into red.

（4）Headache due to liver-yang: Push Qiaogong（along the line from Yifeng（TE 17）to Quepen（ST 12），up to down, twenty times for each side, and do it alternately; sweep by your fingers along the gall bladder meridian from fore-upward to back-downward, alternately for two sides, each side for ten times, and press acupoint of Jiaosun（TE 20）；press and knead Taichong（LR 3），Xingjian（LR 2）till the patient feels sour; rub Yongquan（KI 1）with the palm till it becomes warm.

（5）Headache due to phlegm: Yi zhi chan pushing manipulation on Zhongwan （CV 12），Tianshu（ST 25），each point for one to two minutes; rub the stomach slowly for three minutes; press and knead Pishu（BL20），Weishu（BL 21），Dachang shu（BL 25），Zu Sanli（ST 36），Fenglong（ST 40），Neiguan（PC 6），every point for one minute; rub broadwise quickly by your palm on the left side of the back till the skin becomes much warmer.

（6）Headache due to blood-deficiency: Rub the abdomen slowly for five minutes, especially around the points of Zhongwan（CV 12），Qihai（CV6），Guanyuan（CV 4），rub Governor meridian of the back quickly by your palm till the skin becomes warmer; press and knead Xinshu（BL 15），Keshu（BL17），Zu Sanli（ST 36），Sanyin Jiao（SP 6）till the patient feels a little sour.

（7） Headache due to kidney-deficiency： Rub the abdomen slowly for five minutes, especially around the points of Qihai (CV 6), Guanyuan (CV 4); rub govenor vessel of the back quickly by your palm, and rub broadwise Shenshu (BL 23), Mingmenshu (GV 4) and lumbosacral portion till the skin becomes warmer.

（8） Headache due to blood-stasis: Press Taiyang (EX-HN5) and Cuanzhu (BL 2), each point for one minute; rub forehead and the two sides of gall bladder meridian of the head for three to five times; rub forehead and the areas around the two Taiyang (EX-HN5) till the skin becomes warmer.

六、注意事项

（1）引起头痛的原因较为复杂，推拿虽对缓解头痛症状有较好疗效，但治疗时必须审证求因，按治病务必求其本的原则辨证论治。

（2）推拿治疗头痛时，手法应轻柔，尤其应避免在头面部使用暴力和蛮力，以避免造成医源性损伤。

（3）头痛患者应避免过度劳累，保持情绪稳定，饮食宜清淡。

（4）应加强锻炼，增强体质，并积极治疗原发疾病。

Ⅵ. Notes

（1） The cause of headache is complicated. Although tuina has a good effect on relieving symptoms of headache, the treatment must be based on the differentiating patterns and identifying the etiology. And we must treat the disease with syndrome differentiation by the principle of seeking the root.

（2） When tuina is applied to treat headache, the manipulation must be soft. And avoid applying too much strength on head and face in case of iatrogenic injury.

（3） The patient with headache must avoid overstrain. Keep a stable mood and have a light diet.

（4） The patient needs more exercise to improve his health, and the primary disease should be treated actively.

第五节 失 眠
Section Five   Insomnia

一、概念

失眠是指以经常不能获得正常睡眠为特征的一种病证。轻者入眠困难，或眠而不酣，时寐时醒，醒后不能再寐，严重者可整夜不眠。古代称为"不得寐"或"不寐"。本症可单独出现,也可以与头痛、眩晕、心悸、健忘等症同时出现。多见于西医的神经官能症和围绝经期综合征等。

Ⅰ. Definition

Insomnia, anciently named inability to acquire sleep or sleeplessness, is a disorder which is characterized by frequent inability to acquire normal sleep. In mild cases, the patient finds it hard to fall asleep, or difficult to sleep soundly, or in other words, he/she can't sleep again after waking up. In serious cases, the patient cannot fall asleep all the night. This disorder may occur alone or together with other disorders like headache, vertigo, palpitation, amnesia and so on. In Western medicine, insomnia is usually involved in neurosis, perimenopause syndrome, etc.

二、病因病机

中医认为失眠与心脾两虚、阴虚火旺、痰热内扰和肝郁化火有关。

西医认为失眠的发生与多种因素有关。精神因素是诱发失眠的重要原因。此外,遗传因素、过度疲劳及其他躯体疾病等也可与发病有关。

Ⅱ. Etiology and Pathology

According to Chinese medicine, insomnia is related to dual vacuity of the heart and spleen, *Yin* vacuity with effulgent fire, phlegm-heat harassing the inner body and liver depression transforming into fire.

In Western medicine, the occurrence of insomnia is related to various kinds of factors, among which mental factor is an important reason inducing it. In addition, genetic factor, over fatigue and other physical diseases may also be involved with the onset of insomnia.

三、辨证分型

(1) 心脾两虚:多梦易醒,心悸健忘,神疲乏力,饮食无味,面色少华,舌淡苔薄,脉弱。

(2) 阴亏火旺:心烦失眠,头晕耳鸣,口干津少,五心烦热,舌质红,脉细数,或有梦遗,健忘,心悸,腰酸等证。

(3) 痰热内扰:失眠,胸闷头重,心烦口苦,目眩,苔腻而黄,脉滑数。

(4) 肝郁化火:失眠,性情急躁易怒,不思饮食,口渴喜饮,目赤口苦,小便黄赤,大便秘结,苔黄,脉弦而数。

Ⅲ. Pattern Differentiation

(1) Dual vacuity of the heart and spleen: It is characterized by profuse dreaming,

tendency to wake up easily from sleep, palpitation, forgetfulness, fatigued spirit and lack of strength, experiencing food as lacking in flavor, lusterless facial complexion, pale tongue and thin tongue fur, and weak pulse.

（2）*Yin* vacuity with effulgent fire: It is characterized by heart vexation, sleeplessness, dizziness, tinnitus, dry mouth with scant liquid, vexing heat in the five hearts, red tongue and fine rapid pulse, or dream emission, forgetfulness, palpitation, aching lumbus, etc.

（3）Phlegm-heat harassing the inner body: It is characterized by insomnia, oppression in the chest, heavy-headedness, heart vexation, bitter taste in the mouth, dizzy vision, yellow slimy tongue fur, as well as slippery and rapid pulse.

（4）Liver depression transforming into fire: It is characterized by insomnia, irritability, anorexia, thirst and preference for drinking, reddish eyes, bitter taste in the mouth, yellowish or reddish urine, constipation, reddish tongue, yellow tongue fur, as well stringlike pulse and rapid pulse.

四、诊断要点

（1）有睡眠障碍史。
（2）轻者入寐困难或睡而易醒，醒后难以再眠，重者彻夜难眠。
（3）常伴有头痛、头昏、心悸健忘、神疲乏力、心神不宁、多梦等。
（4）经各系统检查及实验室检查，未发现有妨碍睡眠的其他器质性疾病。

Ⅳ. Diagnostic Points

（1）The patient has a history of sleep disorder.

（2）In mild cases, the patient has difficulty falling asleep, or has liability to wake up during sleep and can't sleep again after waking up. In serious cases, the patient cannot fall asleep all the night.

（3）The disorder often occur together with headache, dizziness, palpation, forgetfulness, disquieted heart spirit, profuse dreaming, etc.

（4）On every systematic examination and laboratory examination no other organic diseases are found to interrupt sleep.

五、推拿治疗

1. 治疗原则

养心安神。虚证辅以健脾滋阴养血，实证则佐以疏肝清热化痰。

2. 部位及穴位

印堂、神庭、睛明、攒竹、太阳、角孙、风池、心俞、肝俞、脾俞、胃俞、肾俞、命门等穴。

3. 手法

一指禅推、揉、抹、按、扫散、拿、滚等法。

4. 基本操作

(1) 患者坐位。医生以一指禅推法或鱼际揉法，从印堂开始向上至神庭，往返 5—6 次；再从印堂向两侧沿眉弓至太阳穴往返 5—6 次；一指禅推眼眶周围，往返 3—4 次；再从印堂沿鼻两侧向下经迎香沿颧骨，至两耳前，往返 2—3 次；治疗过程中以印堂、神庭、睛明、攒竹、太阳穴为重点。

(2) 分抹前额 3—5 次，抹时配合按睛明、鱼腰穴。

(3) 扫散头两侧胆经循行部位，并配合按角孙穴。

(4) 五指拿法从头顶开始，拿到枕骨下部转用三指拿法，并配合拿风池，2—3 分钟。

(5) 患者俯卧位。医生以滚法作用于背腰部，重点在心俞、肝俞、脾俞、胃俞、肾俞、命门穴，3—5 分钟。

(6) 一指禅推或按揉心俞、肝俞、脾俞、胃俞、肾俞、命门穴，每穴 1—2 分钟。

5. 辨证加减

(1) 心脾两虚：按揉心俞、肝俞、胃俞、小肠俞、足三里穴，每穴 1 分钟；掌擦法横擦左侧背部及直擦背部督脉，以透热为度。

(2) 阴虚火旺：推桥弓穴：先推一侧桥弓 20—30 次，再推另一侧桥弓穴；掌擦法先横擦肾俞、命门穴，再擦两侧涌泉穴，以透热为度。

(3) 痰热内扰：按揉中脘、气海、天枢、神门、足三里、丰隆穴，每穴 1 分钟；掌擦法横擦左侧背部及八髎穴，以透热为度。

(4) 肝郁化火：按揉肝俞、胆俞、期门、章门、太冲穴，每穴 1—2 分钟；搓两胁，由上至下，1—2 分钟。

Ⅴ. Tuina Treatment

1. Principle

Nourish the heart and quiet the spirit, with vacuity pattern supported by splenic fortification, enriching yin and nourishing blood, as well as repletion pattern assisted by coursing the liver, clearing heat and transforming phlegm.

2. Acupoints and Location

Yintang (EX-HN 3), Shenting (GV 24), Jingming (BL 1), Cuanzhu(BL 2), Taiyang (EX-HN5), Jiaosun (TE 20), Fengchi (GB 20), Xinshu (BL 15), Ganshu (BL 18), Pishu (BL 20), Weishu (BL 21), Shenshu (BL 23), Mingmen (GV 4), etc.

3. Manipulations

Yi zhi chan pushing, kneading, wiping, pressing, sweeping, grasping, rolling manipulation etc.

4. Basic Manipulations

(1) The patient takes a seating position. The doctor applies Yi zhi chan pushing manipulation or kneading with thenar eminence from Yintang (EX-HN 3) up to Shenting (GV 24) back and forth for 5 to 6 times; then pushes from Yintang (EX-HN 3) to Taiyang (EX-HN 5) along the eyebrows back and forth for 5 to 6 times. Push the orbit with one-finger qi concentration back and forth for 3 to 4 times; then push from Yintang (EX-HN 3) along both sides of the nose, down through Yingxiang (LI 20) along the cheekbone then to the front of both ears, repeat 2 to 3 times. Yintang (EX-HN 3), Shenting (GV 24), Jingming (BL 1), Cuanzhu (BL 2) and Taiyang (EX-HN 5) should be focused during the whole process of manipulation.

(2) Wipe the forehead separately for 3 to 5 times, cooperated with pressing Jingming (BL 1) and Yuyao (EX-HN4).

(3) Sweep out the bilateral courses of the gallbladder meridian, in coordination with pressing Jiaosun (TE 20).

(4) Grasp with five fingers from vertex and then with three fingers to the occipital bone, cooperated with grasping Fengchi (GB 20) for about 2 to 3 minutes.

(5) The patient takes a prone position. The doctor applies rolling on the back, concentrating on Xinshu (BL 15), Ganshu (BL 18), Pishu (BL 20), Weishu (BL 21), Shenshu (BL 23) and Mingmen (GV 4), for about 3 to 5 minutes.

(6) Push with one-finger qi concentration or knead Xinshu (BL 15), Ganshu (BL 18), Pishu (BL 20), Weishu (BL 21), Shenshu (BL 23) and Mingmen (GV 4). Each acupoint takes 1 to 2 minutes.

5. Dialectical Addition and Subtraction

(1) Dual vacuity of the heart and spleen: Press and knead Xinshu (BL 1), Ganshu (BL 18), Weishu(BL 21), Xiaochangshu (BL 27) and Zu Sanli (ST 36), 1 minute for each acupoint; rub the left side of the back horizontally and the governing vessel vertically until it is warm in the local area.

(2) Yin vacuity with effulgent fire: Push Qiaogong on the one side for 20 to 30 minutes, then the other side; rub Shenshu (BL 23) and Mingmen (GV 4) horizontally, and Yongquan (LI 1) until it is warm in the local area.

(3) Phlegm-heat harassing the inner body: Press and knead Zhongwan (CV 12), Qihai (CV 6), Tianshu (ST 25), Shenmen (HT 7), Zu Sanli (ST 36) and Fenglong (ST 40), 1 minute for each acupoint; horizontally rub the left side of the back and Baliao acupoint until it is warm in the local area.

(4) Liver depression transforming into fire: Press and knead Ganshu (BL 18), Danshu (BL 19), Qimen (LR 14), Zhangmen (LR 13) and Taichong (LR 3), 1 to 2 minutes for each acupoint; rub hypochondriac region with the palm up and down for

about 1 minute.

六、注意事项

消除思想顾虑,避免情绪激动;睡前不吸烟、不喝酒和浓茶等东西;养成良好的生活习惯,每天参加适当体力劳动;多参加体育锻炼,增强体质;推拿治疗失眠选择晚上临睡前则效果更佳。

Ⅵ. Notes

Eliminate concerns and avoid rage. Avoid smoking, drinking alcohol or tea before bed time. Develop healthy life habits and do some physical work and exercises every day appropriately. Do some physical work and exercises to strengthen the body. The effect of tuina therapy to treat insomnia right before getting to bed is much better.

第六节 中风后遗症
Section Six Stroke Sequel

一、概念

中风后遗症是指脑血管意外后遗留的一侧肢体瘫痪、偏身麻木、口眼歪斜、言语謇涩或失语等为主要表现的一种临床病证,又称半身不遂、偏枯、偏瘫等,多见于中老年人,大多数人有高血压或心脏病病史。本病一年四季均可发病,但以冬春两季为高发季节。

Ⅰ. Definition

Stroke sequel is a clinical disease, also called hemiplegia, which is a sequel of cerebral vascular accident. The major symptoms are one side of the limb paralysis, hemianesthesia, deviated eyes and mouth, inarticulateness or aphasia, particularly among older people and those who has a history of hypertension or heart disease. This disease could occur in every season but more frequently in winter and spring.

二、病因病机

中医认为本病的病因是由于脏腑功能失调、正气虚弱、情志过极、劳倦内伤、饮食不节、气候骤变等因素,致瘀血阻滞、痰热内生、心火亢盛、肝阳上亢、肝风内动、风火相煽、气血逆乱,上冲于脑而发本病。

西医认为本病是脑血管意外引起的后遗症,脑血管意外分出血性和缺血性两大类,前者包括脑出血和蛛网膜下腔出血,后者包括脑血柱形成和脑栓塞。

Ⅱ. Etiology and Pathology

In Chinese medicine that the basic mechanism is that the factors such as insufficiency of zang-fu organs, deficiency of vital qi, emotional disturbance, over-exertion, improper diet, sudden changes of climate could lead to stagnation of blood stasis, phlegm-heat attacking internally, heart-fire hyperactivity, liver-yang hyperactivity, liver-wind stirring. Wind-yang stirs internally and suddenly. The wind makes qi and blood flow abnormally. When it attacks the brain, there comes stroke sequel.

In Western medicine, stoke sequel is considered as a sequel of cerebral vascular accident. Cerebral vascular accident can be divided into two types: ischemic stroke and hemorrhagic stroke. The former includes cerebral hemorrhage and subarachnoid hemorrhage, the later includes the formation of cerebral blood column and cerebral embolism.

三、临床表现

半身不遂，以单侧上下肢瘫痪无力为主，伴肌肤不仁；初期患者肢体软弱无力，知觉迟钝或稍有强硬，活动功能受限，以后逐渐趋于强直挛急，患侧肢体姿势常发生改变和畸形等；口眼歪斜、舌强语涩或失语等。

Ⅲ. Clinical Manifestations

Hemiplegia, mainly one side of the limb paralysis, along with hemianesthesia. Patients in early stages might feel their limbs physically weak and feeble, dull or even stiff. Their movement is limited, followed by myoclonic jerks, and spasm. The posture of limbs of the affected side often changes and deforms. Facial paralysis, inarticulateness or aphasia are often accompanied.

四、诊断要点

（1）有脑血管意外的病史。

（2）单侧上下肢瘫痪无力、口眼歪斜、舌强语蹇等。

（3）鼻唇沟变浅、口角下垂、表情肌麻痹，不能吹口哨及鼓腮。

（4）患侧肌力减退，感觉减退或消失。

（5）深反射（肱二头肌反射、肱三头肌反射、桡骨膜反射、膝反射、踝反射等）亢进，浅反射（腹壁反射、提睾反射等）减退。

（6）病理反射（巴宾斯基征、霍夫曼征等）阳性，髌阵挛引出。

（7）头颅 CT 检查：出血性，可见脑实质内高密度病灶；缺血性，可见脑实质内低密度病灶。

（8）头颅 MRI 检查：对脑栓塞患者可清晰显示早期缺血性梗死、脑干及小脑梗死、静脉窦血栓形成等，对脑出血患者可发现 CT 不能确定的脑干或小脑少量出血。

（9）数字减影脑血管造影：可检出脑动脉瘤、脑动静脉畸形和血管炎等。

Ⅳ. Diagnostic Points

（1）The patient has a history of cerebral vascular accident.

（2）One side of the limb paralysis, hemianesthesia, deviated eyes and mouth, inarticulateness or aphasia.

（3）Shallow nasolabial groove, prolapsed mouth, and paralyzed facial muscles that the patient could not whistle or bulge his/her cheek.

（4）Weakened muscle force of the affected side, reduced or disappeared sensation.

（5）Exaggeration of the deep reflexes (biceps reflex, triceps reflex, radial menbrane reflex, knee reflex, ankle reflex), and decrease of the superficial reflexes (abdominal reflexes, cremasteric reflexes, etc.)

（6）Positive of the pathological reflexes (Babinski sign, Hoffmann sign, etc.), and appearance of patella clonus.

（7）Skull CT examination: Hypertensity focus is shown on brain parenchyma in ischemic stroke, and low density focus is shown on brain parenchyma in hemorrhagic stroke.

（8）Skull MRI examination: To cerebral embolism patients, cerebral ischemic infarction in early stage, infarction in brainstem and cerebellar and cerebral venous sinus thrombosis could be displayed clearly. To cerebral hemorrhage patients, minor hemorrhage in brainstem or cerebellum couldn't be determined.

（9）Digital subtraction angiogram (DSA): Cerebral aneurysm, cerebral arteriovenous malformation and vasculitis can be detected.

五、推拿治疗

1. 治疗原则

平肝息风、行气活血、舒筋通络、滑利关节。本病以早期治疗为主，一般在中风后两周，且血压稳定后可行推拿治疗。

2. 部位及穴位

背部脊柱两侧膀胱经、颈项两侧和患侧上、下肢，天宗、肝俞、胆俞、膈俞、肾俞、环跳、阳陵泉、委中、承山、风市、伏兔、膝眼、解溪、臂臑、尺泽、曲池、手三里、合谷、太阳、睛明、角孙、风池、风府、肩井等穴。

3. 手法

㨰、按、揉、搓、擦、拿、捻、摇、抹、扫散等法。

4. 基本操作

（1）患者俯卧位。医生站立在病人旁用按揉法作用于背部脊柱两侧膀胱经第一侧线，自上而下 2—3 遍，重点在天宗、肝俞、胆俞、膈俞、肾俞等穴，约 5 分钟。

（2）㨰脊柱两侧，并向下至臀部、股后部、小腿后部。以腰椎两侧、环跳、委中、承山及跟腱部为重点治疗部位，并配合腰后伸和患肢后伸的被动活动，约 5 分钟；横擦腰骶部，以透热为度。

（3）患者仰卧位。医生以㨰法作用于患侧下肢，自髂前上棘向下沿大腿前面，向下至膝关节及足背部治疗，重点在伏兔、膝眼、解溪。同时配合髋关节、膝关节、踝关节的被动伸屈活动和整个下肢的内旋动作，约 5 分钟。

（4）拿患侧下肢、委中、承山，以大腿内侧中部及膝部周围为重点治疗，2—3 分钟；搓下肢，自上而下 2—3 遍。

（5）患者侧卧位。医生以㨰法作用于下肢外侧面，由上而下，3—4 分钟，按揉居髎、风市、阳陵泉、解溪穴，每穴 1 分钟。

（6）患者坐位。医生以㨰法作用于患侧肩部周围及颈项两侧，并配合患肢向背后回旋上举及肩关节外展内收的被动活动，3—5 分钟；㨰法自患侧上臂内侧至前臂进行治疗，以肘关节及其周围为重点治疗部位。在施行㨰法的同时配合肘关节伸屈的被动活动，3—5 分钟；㨰患肢腕部，手掌和手指，同时配合腕关节及指间关节伸屈的被动活动，2—3 分钟。

（7）按揉尺泽、曲池、手三里、合谷等穴，2—3 分钟；捻手指关节，每个手指 3 遍。

（8）拿法自肩部至腕部，往返 3—4 次；摇肩、肘、腕关节，顺、逆时针各 3 遍；搓法自肩部至腕部，往返 2—3 遍。

（9）抹法自印堂至太阳分抹，往返 4—5 遍，同时配合按揉睛明、太阳各 30 次；扫散法在头侧胆经循行部位自前上方向后下方操作，每侧 20—30 次，配合按揉角孙 30 次。

（10）按揉颈项两侧和风池、风府、肩井穴，2—3 分钟；拿风池、肩井各 20—30 次。

5. 随症加减

口眼歪斜可参照面瘫治疗方法。

Ⅴ. Tuina treatment

1. Principle

Calm liver-wind, promote flow of qi and blood circulation to dredge blocked channels, lubricate joints. Early treatment is recommended, tuina therapy can be applied on patients in two weeks after stoke when the blood pressure is stable.

2. Acupoint and Location

Bladder meridian on both sides of the spine on the back, both sides of the neck, limbs of the attracted side, Tianzong (SI 11), Ganshu (BL 18), Danshu (BL 19), Geshu (BL 17), Shenshu (BL 23), Huantiao (GB 30), Yang Lingquan (GB 34), Weizhong (BL 40), Chengshan (BL 57), Fengshi (GB 31), Futu (ST 32), Xiyan (LE 05), Jiexi (ST 41), Binao (LI 14), Chize (LU 05), Quchi (LI 11), Shou Sanli (LI 10), Hegu (LI 4), Taiyang (EX-HN5), Jingming (BL 1), Jiaosun (TE 20), Fengchi (GB 20), Fengfu (GV 16), Jianjing (GB 21).

3. Manipulation

Rolling, pressing, kneading, foulaging, scrubbing, grasping, twirling, rotating, wiping , sweeping manipulation etc.

4. Operation

(1) Patient takes prone position, while the doctor stands beside him, and pushes along the first lateral line of the bladder meridian on the sides of the spinous processes of vertebrae from top to bottom for 2 to 3 times, about 5 minutes in total. Tianzong (SI 11), Ganshu (BL 18), Danshu (BL 19), Geshu (BL 17), Shenshu (BL 23) are the main acupoints in this line.

(2) Roll along both sides of the spine down to the hips, the back of the thighs and the shanks. Treatment focuses on both sides of the lumbar spine, Huantiao (GB 30), Weizhong (BL 40), Chengshan (BL 57), and the achilles tendon. Along with passive activities like backward extension of lumbar spine and limbs gently for 5 minutes, horizontally scrub the lumbosacral portion till it is warm.

(3) For the patient in supine position, the doctor rolls the lower limb from the anterior superior spine along the front of thighs down to knee joint and the dorsum of foot. And the treatment focuses on Futu (ST 32), Xiyan(LE 05) and Jiexi (ST 41). Passive activities such as backward extension of the hip joint, the knee-joint and the ankle joint, and the internal rotation of lower limbs should be coordinated gently for 5 minutes.

(4) Grasp the lower limbs of the affected side, Weizhong (BL 40) and Chengshan (BL 57). The focus of the treatment is the middle part of the inner thighs and the area around the knee. Operate gently from top to bottom for 2 to 3 times.

(5) The patient should be posed at lateral position. The doctor rolls the outer of the lower limb from top to bottom gently for 3 to 4 minutes. Then press and knead Juliao (GB 29), Fengshi (GB 31), Yang Lingquan (GB 34) and Jiexi (ST 41), 1 minute for each acupoint.

(6) With the patient sitting erect, the doctor stands behind him, and rolls the shoulder portion of the affected side and both sides of the neck, along with the passive activities like backward rotation of the upper limb, outreach and adduction of the shoulders, for 3 to 5 minutes. The rolling manipulation should be applied from the

inner side of the upper arms to forearms, and the manipulation should focus on the portion of elbow joint. At the same time, passive activities of bending the elbow forward and backward should be preceded for 3 to 5 minutes. While rolling the wrist, palm and fingers, a passive activity of bending the wrist joint and interphalangeal joint forward and backward is needed at the same time for 2 to 3 minutes.

(7) Press and knead Chize (LU 05), Quchi (LI 11), Shou Sanli (LI 10) and Hegu (LI 4) for 2 to 3 minutes. Twirl the finger joints 3 times for each.

(8) Grasp from the shoulder to the wrist 3 to 4 times back and forth. Then rotate the shoulder joint, elbow joint and wrist joint 3 times clockwise and 3 time anticlockwise. Foulage from the shoulder to wrist 2 or 3 times back and forth.

(9) Wipe from Yintang (EX-HN 3) to Taiyang (EX-HN5) (both in the same side) 4 to 5 time back and forth, along with pressing and kneading Jingming (BL 1) and Taiyang (EX-HN5) 30 times for each. Sweep out along the gallbladder meridian from the anterior upper side to the posterior lower side, 20 to 30 times for each side, along with pressing and kneading Jiaosun (TE 20) for 30 times.

(10) Press and knead both sides of the neck, Fengchi (GB 20), Fengfu (GV 16) and Jianjing (GB 21) about 2 to 3 minutes, and grasp Fengchi (GB 20) and Jianjing (GB 21) 20 to 30 times for each acupoint.

5. Modification According to Symptoms

Patients with deviated eyes and mouth can be treated with the method operating on patient with facial paralysis.

六、注意事项

(1) 推拿治疗中风后遗症效果较满意。且本病病程的长短与瘫痪肢体的康复有直接关系,故应尽早对本病进行治疗,一般在中风后两周,且血压稳定后可行推拿治疗。

(2) 推拿治疗本病时手法宜轻柔,被动活动手法应在病人能忍受范围内进行,防止医源性损伤。

(3) 应鼓励患者在接受推拿治疗的同时,积极进行自我功能的康复锻炼,并预防压疮、尿路感染、坠积性肺炎等。

(4) 推拿对 1—2 年以上病程的中风后遗症,收效甚微。

Ⅵ. Notes

(1) Therapeutic effects of Tuina therapy in stoke sequel are satisfactory. Since its duration is directly related to the recovery of the affected limbs, patients should be treated as soon as possible. In general, tuina therapy can be used on patients in two weeks after stoke when the blood pressure is stable.

（2） The manipulation should be applied in a gentle way. The application of passive activities should be under the endurance of patients to prevent iatrogenic injuries.

（3） We should encourage patients to take actively functional rehabilitation exercise along with Tuina therapy. And prevent decubital ulcer, urinary tract infection, and hypostatic pneumonia as well.

（4） Tuina therapy in patients with a 1 or 2 years history of stoke sequel has less effect.

第九章 小儿常见病的推拿治疗
Chapter Nine Tuina Treatment for Common Diseases in Children

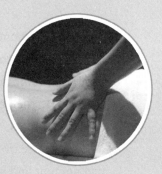

第一节 腹 泻
Section One Diarrhea

一、概念

婴儿腹泻亦名消化不良,是以腹泻为主要症状的一种常见病。本病四季皆可发生,而尤以夏、秋两季为多。如治疗不及时,迁延日久可影响小儿的营养、生长和发育。重症患儿还可产生脱水、酸中毒等一系列严重症状,甚至危及生命。

现代医学根据腹泻之轻重将其分为轻型(单纯性消化不良)和重型(中毒性消化不良)。重型者临床症状皆较重,并伴有显著的全身症状,可由轻型转变而来,亦可急性发病,腹泻一般每天 10 次以上,粪便中含大量水分,患儿食欲缺乏、并常并发呕吐、发热等,体重很快下降,若不及时治疗,可逐渐出现脱水和酸中毒的症状,甚至可危及生命,故在临床上必须严密观察病情变化。

本病证属西医学消化不良、小儿肠炎、秋季腹泻、肠功能紊乱等疾病。

Ⅰ. Definition

Infantile diarrhea is also called indigestion, which is a common disease with diarrhea as main symptom. The disease can occur in all seasons, especially in summer and autumn. If the treatment is not timely, long-time procrastination can affect the growth, development and nutrition of infant. In severe cases, they will also get dehydration, acidosis and a series of serious symptoms, or even endanger their life.

Modern medicine, according to the severity of diarrhea, divides it into mild (simple indigestion) and severe (toxic indigestion). The latter one's clinical symptoms are serious, associated with a significant systemic symptoms. It can be transformed from the mild one, and can be also acutely attacked. A patient with diarrhea defecates generally more than 10 times a day, with feces containing large amounts of water, low appetite, vomiting and fever, so his weight tends to decrease quickly. Without timely treatment，the patient can emerge the symptoms of dehydration and acidosis, and even face life threats. Therefore, the patient's condition must be closely observed.

This disease equals to indigestion, child enteritis, autumn diarrhea, bowel dysfunction and so on in Western Medicine.

二、病因病机

中医认为婴儿腹泻的发生与下列因素有关：

（1）感受外邪：腹泻的发生与气候有密切关系。寒、湿、暑、热之邪皆能引起腹泻，而尤以湿邪引起的为多。脾恶湿喜燥、湿困脾阳，使运化不健,对饮食水谷的消化、吸收发生障碍而致腹泻。

（2）内伤乳食：由于喂养不当、饥饱无度,或突然改变食物性质,或感食油腻、生冷,或饮食不洁,导致脾胃损伤、运化失职、不能腐熟水谷而致除泻。

（3）脾胃虚弱：小儿脏腑娇嫩,脾常不足,且小儿生机蓬勃,脾胃负担相对较重,一旦遇到外来因素的影响就能导致脾胃受损,使水谷不得运化,则水反而为湿,谷反而为滞,水湿滞留,下注肠道而为腹泻。

现代医学认为婴儿腹泻除与饮食、气候等因素有关外,尚与致病性大肠杆菌、病毒及其他感染有关。

Ⅱ. Etiology and Pathology

Traditional Chinese medicine believes that the occurrence of infantile diarrhea is related to the following factors:

（1）Contracting the external evil: The occurrence of diarrhea is closely related to climate. Cold, wet, summer heat, heat evil can all cause diarrhea, especially the dampness. Spleen dislikes dampness and prefers dry. If dampness troubles spleen yang, the transportation can't work well, troubling digestion and absorption of grain and water, leading to diarrhea.

（2）Hurt internally by infantile food: Due to improper diet, excessive hunger or a sudden change of the nature of the food, or eating greasy, raw or cold food; or having a unclean diet, can result in damage to the spleen and stomach, whose transportation and dereliction duty cannot be well played, unable to decompose grain and water, leading to diarrhea.

（3）Deficiency of spleen and stomach: Children's viscera are delicate and spleen is often deficient. In addition, infants are in growth, so that spleen and stomach are taking a relative heavy burden. Once they are influenced by some factors, their spleen and stomach will be hurt, leading to grain and water not being digested, then water turns into dampness, and dampness retention will go down to bowel, leading to diarrhea.

Modern medicine believes that baby diarrhea, in addition to diet, climate and other factors, is related to pathogenic *Escherichia coli*, viruses and other infections.

三、诊断和鉴别诊断

1. 诊断要点

（1）大便次数增多，每日 3—5 次或多达 10 次以上，色淡黄，如蛋花汤样，或色褐而臭，可有少量黏液，或伴有恶心、呕吐、腹痛、发热、口渴等症。

（2）有乳食不节、饮食不洁或感受时邪病史。

（3）重者泄泻及呕吐较严重，可见小便短少、体温升高、烦渴神萎、皮肤干瘪、囟门凹陷、目眶下陷、啼哭无泪、口唇樱红、呼吸深长及腹胀等症。

（4）大便镜检可有脂肪球或少量红细胞、白细胞。

（5）大便病原体检查可见致病性大肠杆菌生长，或分离出轮状病毒等病原体。

2. 实验室检查

（1）大便镜检可有脂肪球或少量红细胞、白细胞。

（2）大便病原体检查可见致病性大肠杆菌生长，或分离出轮状病毒等病原体。

3. 鉴别诊断

痢疾：痢疾初起大便稀、便次增多、腹痛明显、里急后重，大便有黏冻、脓血。大便培养有痢疾杆菌生长。

III. Diagnosis and Differential Diagnosis

1. Essentials of Diagnosis

（1）The frequency of defecation increases from 3 – 5 times a day or up to more than 10 times, with yellow stool like egg flower soup, or brown and smelly. In addition, stool can be with a small amount of mucus, or the patient will be accompanied by diseases like nausea, vomiting, abdominal pain, fever, thirst, and so on.

（2）The patient has a medical history of unclean infantile food, dirty diet or getting external evil.

（3）In serious cases, the patients have severe diarrhea and vomiting, and oliguresis can be seen, with symptoms like elevated body temperature, bored, polydipsia and low spirit, dry skin, sunken fontanel, sunken eye socket, crying without tears, cherry lips red, deep breathing and abdominal distention.

(4) A small amount of fat ball or red blood cells, white blood cells can be found in stool examination.

(5) The growth of pathogenic *Escherichia coli* can be seen, or rotavirus and other pathogens can be isolated in fecal pathogens examination.

2. Laboratory Examination

(1) A small amount of fat ball or red blood cells, white blood cells can be found in stool examination.

(2) The growth of pathogenic *Escherichia coli* can be seen, or rotavirus and other pathogens can be isolated in fecal pathogens examination.

3. Differential Diagnosis

Dysentery: At the beginning of dysentery, the stool is watery with increased frequency of defecation, accompanied with obvious abdomen pain and tenesmus. And stool is sticky and frozen with pus and blood. There is *dysentery bacillus* growth in stool bacteria culture.

四、推拿治疗

1. 辨证分型

（1）寒湿泻：大便清稀多沫、色淡不臭，肠鸣腹痛，面色淡白，口不渴，小便清长，苔白腻，脉濡，指纹色红。

（2）湿热泻：腹痛即泻，急迫暴注，色黄褐热臭，身有微热，口渴，尿少色黄，苔黄腻，脉滑数，指纹色紫。

（3）伤食泻：腹痛胀满，泻前哭闹，泻后痛减，大便量多酸臭，口臭纳呆，或伴呕吐酸馊，苔厚或垢腻，脉滑。

（4）脾虚泻：久泻不愈或经常反复发作，面色苍白，食欲缺乏，便稀夹有奶块及食物残渣，或每于食后即泻，舌淡苔薄，脉濡。

2. 辨证施治

（1）寒湿泻。

治则：温中散寒，化湿止泻。

处方：补脾经、推三关、补大肠、揉外劳、揉脐、推上七节骨、揉龟尾、按揉足三里。

方义：推三关、揉外劳温阳散寒，配补脾经、揉脐按揉足三里能健脾化湿，温中散寒；补大肠、推上七节骨、揉龟尾温中止泻。

（2）湿热泻。

治则：清热利湿，调中止泻。

处方：清脾胃、清大肠、清小肠、退六腑、揉天枢、揉龟尾。

方义：清脾胃以清中焦湿热；清大肠、揉天枢清利肠府湿热积滞；退六腑、清小肠清热利尿除湿；配揉龟尾以理肠止泻。

（3）伤食泻。

治则：消食导滞，和中助运。

处方：补脾经、清大肠、揉板门、运内八卦、揉中脘、摩腹、揉天枢、揉龟尾。

方义：补脾经、揉中脘、运内八卦、揉板门、摩腹健脾和胃，行滞消食；清大肠、揉天枢疏调肠府积滞；配揉龟尾以理肠止泻。

（4）脾虚泻。

治则：健脾益气，温阳止泻。

处方：补脾经、补大肠、推三关、摩腹、揉脐、推上七节骨、揉龟尾、捏脊。

方义：补脾经、补大肠健脾益气，固肠实便；推三关、摩腹、揉脐、捏脊温阳补中；配推上七节骨、揉龟尾以温阳止泻。

Ⅳ. Tuina Treatment

1. Syndrome Differentiation

(1) Cold-dampness diarrhea: watery stool with foam, light color with no stink smell, presence of bowel sounds and abdominal pain, pale white complexion, no thirst, clear abundant urine, white and greasy tongue coating, soggy pulse, red fingers.

(2) Dampness-heat diarrhea: immediate diarrhea with abdominal pain, urgent diarrhea, tan in color with stink smell, feeling slightly hot and thirsty, few urine with yellow color, white and greasy tongue coating, slippery and rapid pulse, purple fingers.

(3) Diarrhea due to improper diet: abdominal pain and fullness, crying and screaming before diarrhea with relieved pain after diarrhea, substantial stool which smells sour and stink, bad breath and poor appetite. Some may be accompanied with vomiting sour food, thick or greasy tongue coating and slippery pulse

(4) Spleen-deficiency diarrhea: chronic unhealed diarrhea or often repeated attacks, pale white complexion, bad appetite, watery stool mixed with milk blocks and food residues, or diarrhea normally occurs

2. Treatment Based on Syndrome Differentiation

(1) Cold-dampness diarrhea

Therapeutic principles: warm the middle energizer to dispel cold, and resolve dampness to cure diarrhea.

Formula: supplement the spleen meridian, manipulate Sanguan, supplement the large intestine, massage Wailao and navel, shove the upper Qijiegu, massage Guiwei and Zu Sanli(ST 36).

Mechanism of prescription: manipulate Sanguan and massage Wailao to warm yang and dispel cold, along with supplementing the spleen meridian to invigorate spleen and eliminate dampness; supplement the large intestine, manipulate the upper

Qijiegu and massage Guiwei to warm the middle energizer and cure diarrhea.

(2) Dampness-heat diarrhea

Therapeutic principle: clear heat and promote diuresis, regulate middle energizer and cure diarrhea.

Formula: clear spleen, stomach, large intestine, small intestine, manipulate Liufu, massage Tianshu (ST 25) and Guiwei.

Mechanism of prescription: clear spleen and stomach to clear the dampness-heat of middle energizer; clear large intestine and massage Tianshu (ST 25) to clear and remove the dampness-heat stagnation of intestines; manipulate Liufu, clear small intestine to clear heat, promote diuresis and eliminate dampness, along with massaging Guiwei to regulate intestines and cure diarrhea.

(3) Improper diet diarrhea

Therapeutic principle: promote digestion and purgation, regulate the middle energizer to help transport.

Formula: supplement the spleen meridian, clear large intestine, massage Banmen, Neibagua and Zhongwan (CV 12), manipulate abdomen, massage Tianshu (ST 25) and Guiwei.

Mechanism of prescription: supplement the spleen meridian, massage Zhongwan (CV 12), Neibagua, Banmen and manipulate abdomen to strength spleen and regulate stomach, promote digestion and consume food; clear large intestine, massage Tianshu (ST 25) to regulate the stagnation of intestines, along with massaging Guiwei to adjust intestines and cure diarrhea.

(4) Spleen-deficiency diarrhea

Therapeutic principle: invigorate spleen and supplement qi, warm yang and cure diarrhea.

Formula: supplement the spleen meridian and large intestine, massage Sanguan, manipulate abdomen, massage navel, upper Qijiegu and Guiwei, chiropractic.

Mechanism of prescription: supplement the spleen meridian and large intestine to invigorate spleen and supplement qi, strength the intestines and solidify stool; manipulate Sanguan and abdomen, massage navel, pinch spine to warm yang and strength the middle energizer, along with manipulating upper Qijiegu and Guiwei to warm yang and cure diarrhea.

五、预防与转归

1. 预防

(1) 注意饮食卫生,不吃不洁食物,防止病从口入。

（2）乳贵有时，食贵有节，做到乳食节制，不要时饥时饱、过凉过热。

（3）泄泻期间，应食宜消化和清淡之品，如奶糕、粥糜等；不食油腻之品。

2. 转归

婴儿腹泻及时正确治疗，则病可痊愈。若不及时治疗或治疗不当，轻者迁延日久，可影响小儿营养、生长和发育，重者可引起严重脱水、代谢性酸中毒、低钾血症而危及生命。

Ⅴ. Prevention and Development

1. Prevention

(1) Pay attention to dietetic hygiene; do not eat contaminated food; prevent disease from entering by the mouth.

(2) It is valuable to feed milk on time and take moderate food. Learn to be temperate in food and milk. Don't be starved or be full, and do not eat food that is too hot or too cold.

(3) During diarrhea, baby should be fed with digestible and light food, such as rice flour and porridge; greasy food is forbidden.

2. Development

Infantile diarrhea, if treated correctly and timely, can be cured. If it is not treated timely or correctly, in mild cases, babies can not be cured for months. Therefore, it may influence infant nutrition, growth and development. In severe cases, babies may have severe dehydration, metabolic acidosis and hypokalemia which can be life-threatening.

第二节　疳　积
Section Two　Malnutrition

一、概念

疳积是疳症和积滞的总称，积滞与疳症有轻重程度的不同。积滞是指小儿伤于乳食，损伤脾胃，而致脾胃运化失司，积聚留滞于中，引起的胃肠疾病，以腹泻或便秘、呕吐、腹胀为主要症状。疳症是由于喂养不当或脾胃受损，影响小儿生长发育的慢性疾病。以小儿面黄肌瘦、头发稀疏、精神疲惫、腹部胀大、青筋暴露或腹凹如舟，饮食异常为主要表现。疳证往往是积滞的进一步发展。积久不消，转化为疳，故有"无积不成疳""积为疳之母"之说。小儿感染诸虫，也可转为疳症。

积滞可见于西医学中的消化功能紊乱，而疳证可见于西医学中的轻、中、重度的小儿营养不良。

Ⅰ. Definition

Infantile malnutrition is the combination of Gan syndrome and Ji syndrome, and the difference between them is the severity of the symptoms. Ji syndrome indicates a kind of infantile gastrointestinal disease. If children take too much food or milk, the spleen and stomach would be hurt, so that they would lose the function of movement and transformation and food would be left in stomach which causes the disease. The main symptom includes diarrhea or constipation, emesis and abdominal distension. Gan syndrome is a kind of chronic disease affecting children's growth and development that results from improper feeding or damaged spleen and stomach. Its main manifestation includes emaciation with sallow complexion, lack of hair, neurolysis, abdominal distension, prominent veins or abdominal retraction and eating disorder. Gan syndrome is usually the further development of Ji syndrome. If Ji syndrome hasn't been treated well, it would develop into Gan syndrome. Thus there are sayings like "there is no Gan without Ji" and "Ji is the mother of Gan". Besides, Gan syndrome can also be caused if children were infected by parasites.

In western medicine, Ji syndrome appears in disorders of digestion and Gan syndrome can be found in light, moderate and severe infantile malnutrition.

二、病因病机

1. 乳食不节、伤及脾胃

脾主运化，胃主受纳，小儿乳食不节，过食肥甘生冷，伤及脾胃，脾胃失司，受纳运化失职。

2. 脾胃虚寒薄弱

脾胃虚寒薄弱，则乳食难于腐熟，而使乳食停积，壅聚中州，阻碍气机，时日渐久，致使营养失调，患儿羸瘦，气液虚衰，发育障碍。

乳食积滞与脾胃虚弱互为因果，积滞可伤及脾胃，脾胃虚弱又能产生积滞，故临床上多互相兼杂为患。此外感染虫症和某些慢性疾病也常为本病的原因。

西医认为有以下原因：长期饮食不当，热量不足；慢性消化性疾病；其他如早产、双胎是导致营养不良的先天条件。较重的营养不良大多是由于多种原因所致。

Ⅱ. Etiology and Pathology

1. Improper Diet Hurting Spleen and Stomach

Spleen governs movement and transformation and stomach receives food and drink. When children have improper diets and take too much fat, sweet, raw, cold food, the spleen and stomach are hurt so as to lose their function of receiving, movement and transformation.

2. Deficiency-cold in Spleen and Stomach

When there is deficiency-cold in spleen and stomach, it will be difficult to digest food and milk, so they will stay in Zhongzhou and stagnate qi. After a period, it will cause malnutrition, thinness and weakness, deficiency of qi and fluid and dysgenopathy.

Milk and food stagnation and weak spleen and stomach interact as both cause and effect. Stagnation may damage spleen and stomach while weak spleen and stomach may cause stagnation, so they usually mix with each other clinically. In addition, infection of parasites and some chronic diseases may also be the pathogenesis.

In western medicine, the reasons are as followed: Long-term imbalance diet, lack of energy and digestive system disease. Premature birth and twins are congenital conditions of malnutrition. Most severe malnutrition is caused by several factors.

三、诊断和鉴别诊断

1. 诊断要点

（1）积滞：乳食不思或少思，脘腹胀痛，呕吐酸馊，大便溏泄，臭如败卵或便秘；烦躁不安，夜间哭闹或发热等症；有伤乳、伤食史；大便检查，有不消化食物残渣或脂肪球。

（2）疳症：饮食异常，大便干稀不调，或脘腹膨胀等明显脾胃功能失调者；形体消瘦，体重低于正常平均值的 15%—40%，面色不华，毛发稀疏枯黄，严重者形体干枯羸瘦，体重可低于正常值 40% 以上；兼有精神不振，或好发脾气，烦躁易怒，或喜揉眉擦眼，或吮指磨牙等症；有喂养不当或病后饮食失调及长期消瘦史；因蛔虫引起者，谓之"蛔疳"，大便镜检可查见蛔虫卵；贫血者，血红蛋白及红细胞计数减少；出现肢体浮肿，属于营养性水肿者，血清总蛋白大多在 45 g/L 以下，血清白蛋白量约在 20 g/L 以下。

2. 鉴别诊断

疳积与消化不良：消化不良即婴儿腹泻，是以腹泻为主要症状。严重的腹泻患儿虽也可伴有食欲缺乏、精神萎靡，但其主证仍为腹泻，故两者可鉴别。

Ⅲ. Diagnosis and Differential Diagnosis

1. Essentials of Diagnosis

（1）Ji syndrome: Lack of appetite, abdominal distention and pain, emesis, diarrhea with rotten eggs smells or constipation. Dysphoria, crying or fever at night, etc. Having a medical history of being hurt by too much milk or food. Presence of indigested food residue or fat globules in stool examination.

（2）Gan syndrome: Obvious spleen and stomach dysfunction such as eating disorder, dry or loose stool disorder, or abdominal distention, emaciation with the weight 15% ~ 40% lower than normal average, lusterless complexion and sparse dry yellow hair. Severe patients are thin and weak and their weight can be more than 40% lower than normal average. Lassitude or often losing one's temper and irritability, or preference to malaxating eyebrow and eyes, or finger sucking and odontoprisis, etc. are often accompanied. Having a medical history of improper feeding or eating disorders after disease and long-term emaciation. Malnutrition with ascariasis is caused by roundworm, and we can see ova of roundworm by microscopic examination of stool. The hemoglobin and erythrocyte of the anemic person is decreased. Limb edema will appear in nutritional edema person whose total serum protein under 45 g/L mostly and the serum albumin level under 20 g/L.

2. Differential Diagnosis

Gan Ji and dyspepsia: Dyspepsia is infantile diarrhea, with the main symptoms of diarrhea. Although severe diarrhea may be associated with poor appetite and drooping spirits, its main syndrome is still diarrhea. Hence, these two diseases can be identified.

四、推拿治疗

1. 辨证分型

（1）积滞伤脾：形体消瘦，体重不增腹部胀满，纳食不香，精神不振，夜寐不安，大便不调常有恶臭，舌苔厚腻。

（2）气血两亏：面色萎黄或㿠白，毛发枯黄稀疏，骨瘦如柴，精神萎靡或烦躁，睡卧不宁，啼声低小，四肢不温，发育障碍，腹部凹陷，大便溏泄，舌淡苔薄，指纹色淡。

2. 辨证施治

（1）积滞伤脾。

治则：消积导滞，调理脾胃。

处方：补脾经、揉板门、推四横纹、运内八卦、揉中脘、分腹阴阳、揉天枢、按揉足三里。

方义：揉板门、揉中脘、分腹阴阳、揉天枢消食导滞，疏调肠胃积滞；推四横纹、运内八卦加强以上作用，并能理气调中；补脾经、按揉足三里以健脾开胃，消食和中。

（2）气血两亏。

治则：温中健脾，补益气血。

处方：补脾经、推三关、揉外劳、掐揉四横纹、运内八卦、揉中脘、按揉足三里、捏脊。

方义：补脾经、推三关、揉中脘、捏脊温中健脾，补益气血，增进饮食；运内八卦、揉外劳温阳助运，理气和血，并加强前四法的作用；掐揉四横纹主治疳积，配按揉足三里调和气血，消导积滞。

Ⅳ. Tuina Treatment

1. Syndrome Differentiation

(1) Indigestion impairing the spleen: emaciation, no increase in weight, abdominal distension, poor appetite, drooping spirits, restless sleep, stool irregularities with rotten, thick and greasy tongue.

(2) Dual depletion of qi and blood: sallow or pale complexion, yellow and sparse hair, skin and bones, drooping spirits, restless sleep, low cry, cold limbs, developmental disorders, abdominal retraction, loose stools, pale and thin tongue, pale fingerprint.

2. Treatment Based on Syndrome Differentiation

(1) Indigestion impairing the spleen

Therapeutic principle: Promote digestion and dispel food stagnation, regulate spleen and stomach.

Formula: Reinforce spleen meridian, massage Banmen, Sihengwen, internal Eight Diagrams, Zhongwan(CV 12), abdominal yin and yang, Tianshu (ST 25), Zu Sanli (ST 36).

Mechanism of prescription: Massaging Banmen, Zhongwan (CV 12), abdominal yin and yang, Tianshu (ST 25) can promote digestion and adjust gastrointestinal accumulation. Massaging Sihengwen, internal Eight Diagrams can enforce the above-mentioned functions and regulate qi. Reinforcing spleen meridian and massaging Zu Sanli (ST 36) can invigorate stomach.

(2) Dual depletion of qi and blood

Therapeutic principle: warm middle and invigorate spleen, tonify qi and blood.

Formula: Reinforce spleen meridian, massage Sanguan, Wailao, Sihengwen, internal Eight Diagrams, Zhongwan (CV 12), Zu Sanli (ST 36) and chiropractics.

Mechanism of prescription: Reinforcing spleen meridian, massage Sanguan, Zhongwan (CV 12), and chiropractics can not only warm middle and invigorate spleen, but also tonify qi and blood and improve diet. Massaging internal Eight Diagrams, Wailao can warm yang and help transportation and regulate the qi and blood, and also enforce the effects of the above. The major functions of massaging Sihengwen is to treat infantile malnutrition, and cooperating with massaging Zu Sanli (ST 36) can regulate qi and blood and promote digestion and remove food retention.

五、预防与转归

1. 预防

防偏食、嗜食、异食,合理喂养;补充营养,增强体质。

2. 转归

疳积之证及早治疗,则一般易治。若防治失时,则迁延日久,累及他脏而缠绵难愈,影响小儿发育。

Ⅴ. Prevention and Development

1. Prevention

Prevent from diet preference, adephagia and parorexia. Feed properly; improve their nutritional intake and physique.

2. Development

It is much easier to treat malnutritional stagnation if the patients go to a doctor as soon as possible. If this disease isn't treated in time and even becomes out of control, it may involve other viscera and become much harder to be cured. And it will influence the development of children as well.

第三节　便　秘
Section Three　Constipation

一、概念

便秘是大便秘结不通,排便时间延长,或欲大便而艰涩不畅的一种病证。本证相当于西医学中由饮食不足、食物成分不适当,肠道功能失常等所致的单纯性便秘。

Ⅰ. Definition

Constipation is a disease with the symptoms of the hard dry stools, the extension of defecation time, or the difficulty to defecate. This disease equals the simple constipation caused by dietary deficiency, improper food composition and intestinal dysfunction in western medicine.

二、病因病机

1. 中医观点

中医认为便秘与饮食不节、燥热、气虚等有关。

饮食不节,过食辛热厚味,以致肠胃积热,气滞不行,或于热病后耗伤津液,导致肠道燥热,津液失于输布而不能下润,于是大便秘结,难于排出。

先天不足,身体虚弱;或病后体虚,气血亏损。气虚则大肠传送无力,血虚则津少不能滋润大肠,以致辞大便排出困难。

2. 西医观点

西医认为便秘的发生有以下原因：

（1）饮食不足：婴儿进食太少时，经过消化后余渣少，大便自然减少。奶中糖量不足，可使大便干燥。

（2）食物成分不适宜：大便性质与食物成分关系密切。

（3）肠道功能失常：由于生活不规律和缺乏训练按时大便的习惯，以致未形成排便的条件反射，终至肠肌松弛而便秘。

（4）体格与生理的缺点：肛门裂、肛门狭窄、先天性巨结肠等都可引起便秘。

（5）精神因素：小儿环境和生活习惯的突然改变，突然的精神刺激等都可引起轻重不等的短时间便秘。

Ⅱ. Etiology and Pathology

1. Traditional Chinese Medicine Opinion

Traditional Chinese medicine considers that constipation is related to eating and drinking without temperance, dryness-heat, deficiency of qi and others.

Both eating and drinking without temperance and having too much spicy or greasy delicious food will cause gastrointestinal heat and stagnation of qi. In addition, body fluids is consumed after heat disease, and it causes dryness-heat in intestinal tract. Body fluids can't transport and moisten the intestinal tract, therefore, the stools become tough and dry and hard to defecate.

Congenitally deficient and weakness, or loss of qi and blood after a disease. Deficiency of qi will reduce the energy of the large intestine to transmit, while the deficiency of blood and body fluids will lower the ability to moisten the large intestine. Both of the two aspects will cause the result that the stools are difficult to be passed out.

2. Western Medicine Opinion

In western medicine, children constipation is caused by following reasons:

（1）Not enough diet: Children's deficiency of diet intake leads to low waste after digestion, definitely, ending up with tiny amount of stool.

（2）Improper diet: Stool texture is closely related to the component of food.

（3）Dysfunction of intestine: People who have poor lifestyles and defecation habits may stop feeling the urge to have bowel movements, eventually leading to the constipation.

（4）Physical defects: Physical diseases, such as anal fissure, anal stenosis and congenital megacolon can cause constipation.

（5）Metal factors: Sudden changes of living environment and lifestyles and sudden mental stimulation may cause short-term constipation with variable degrees of severity.

三、诊断和鉴别诊断

1. 诊断要点

（1）根据患儿大便秘结不通，大便干结、坚硬，便量不多，呈栗子状，偶可伴有少量鲜血。

（2）肛门指检未触及肛门及直肠下端的异物。

（3）X线钡剂灌肠或直肠镜检查，未见因肠管内或肠管外器质性病变引起的肠管堵塞。

2. 鉴别诊断

巨结肠（先天性）：一个月内婴儿便秘并伴有腹胀者，则应考虑是否为本病。肛门指检及X线钡剂灌肠检查能帮助诊断。

Ⅲ. Diagnosis and Differential Diagnosis

1. Essentials of Diagnosis

（1）Bowel movement obstruction, tiny amount of dry and hard stools in the shape of chestnuts, sometimes blood stools

（2）No foreign bodies can be touched on the anus and lower rectum by digital examination of rectum.

（3）Intestinal blockage caused by any intra-intestinal or extra-intestinal organic disease cannot be found by the X-ray barium enema or rectoscope.

2. Differential Diagnosis

Megacolon (congenital): If the baby has constipation and abdominal distension within the first mouth of life, this disease should be taken into consideration. And digital examination of rectum and X-ray barium enema can help the diagnosis.

四、推拿治疗

1. 辨证分型

（1）实秘：大便干结，面赤身热，口臭唇赤，小便短赤，胸胁痞满，纳食减少，腹部胀痛，苔黄燥，指纹色紫。

（2）虚秘：面色㿠白无华，形瘦乏力，神疲气怯，大便努挣难下，舌淡苔薄，指纹色淡。

2. 辨证施治

（1）实秘。

治则：顺气行滞，清热通便。

处方：清大肠、退六腑、运内八卦、按揉膊阳池、摩腹、按揉足三里、推下七节骨、搓摩胁肋、揉天枢。

方义：清大肠、揉天枢荡涤肠府邪热积滞；摩腹、按揉足三里健脾和胃，行滞消食；搓摩胁肋、运内八卦疏肝理气，顺气行滞；按揉膊阳池、推下七节骨配退六腑以通便清热。

（2）虚秘。

治则：益气养血，滋阴润燥。

处方：补脾经、清大肠、推三关、揉上马、按揉膊阳池、按揉足三里、揉肾俞、捏脊。

方义：补脾经、推三关、捏脊、按揉足三里补养气血，健脾调中，强壮身体；清大肠、按揉膊阳池配揉上马、揉脐、揉肾俞滋阴润燥理肠通便。

Ⅳ. Tuina Treatment

1. Syndrome Differentiation

（1）Excessive constipation: dry stools, flushed face with fever sensation in body, halitosis and red lips, scanty deep yellow urine, fullness in the chest and hypochondriac, poor appetite, abdominal distention, yellow and dry coating, and purple fingerprint.

（2）Deficient constipation: pale and lusterless complexion, thinness and fatigue, spiritlessness and timidity, desire to defecate but weakness in trial, pale tongue with thin coating, and pale fingerprint.

2. Treatment Based on Syndrome Differentiation

（1）Excessive constipation

Therapeutic principle: Promote qi circulation and remove stagnation, clear heat and relieve constipation.

Formula: Push Dachangjing; push Liufu; acr-push Neibagua; knead Boyangchi; rub abdomen; knead Zu Sanli (ST 36); push Qijiegu downwards; twist and rub hypochondrium; and knead Tianshu (ST 25).

Mechanism of prescription: Pushing Dachangjing and kneading Tianshu (ST 25) can eliminate the accumulative stagnation and heat in intestine. Rubbing abdomen and kneading Zu Sanli (ST 36) are capable of strengthening spleen and regulating stomach, promoting digestion and removing stagnation. Twisting and rubbing hypochondrium and acr-pushing Neibagua can smooth liver and regulate qi, promote qi circulation and remove stagnation. Kneading Boyangchi and pushing Qijiegu downwards mean to relieve constipation and clear heat.

（2）Deficient constipation

Therapeutic principle: Tonify qi and blood, nourish yin and moisturize dryness.

Formula: Tonify Pijing; push Dachangjing and Sanguan; knead Shangma, Boyangchi, Zu Sanli (ST 36) and Shenshu (BL 23); and pinch spine.

Mechanism of prescription: Tonifying Pijing, pushing Sanguan, pinching spine and kneading Zu Sanli (ST 36) are able to build up body constitution by tonifying qi and blood, strengthening spleen and harmonizing qi of the middle energizer. Pushing Dachangjing, kneading Boyangchi with kneading Shangma, umbilicus and Shenshu (BL 23) can promote bowel movements by nourishing yin and moisturizing dryness.

五、预防与转归

1. 预防

培养按时排便的习惯；宜食带纤维的蔬菜；脾胃虚少食而便少者，应注意抚养胃气。

2. 转归

便秘一般易治，但若由先天性巨结肠引起之便秘，推拿治疗欠佳者必要时可行手术治疗。

Ⅴ. Prevention and Development

1. Prevention

Establishing a regular pattern of defecation; eat more vegetables rich in fiber; for constipation resulting from little intake of food which is caused by the deficiency of spleen and stomach, strengthening stomach qi should be the focus to relieve constipation.

2. Development

Generally speaking, constipation is an easily treatable disease. However, for the constipation caused by congenital megacolon and responding poorly to Tuina therapy, if necessary, operation should be taken.

第四节　发　热
Section Four　Fever

一、概念

发热即体温异常升高，是小儿常见的一种病证。临床上一般可分为外感发热、肺胃实热、阴虚内热三种。外感发热，一般是指感冒而言，但急性传染病初起时也可见到，对于年幼体弱小儿，由于得病以后容易出现兼症，应予注意。

本节仅叙述由上呼吸道感染而引起的某些急性发热和部分功能性发热。

Ⅰ. Definition

Fever, a common symptom in pediatrics, is a condition of abnormal high body temperature. In general, it can be divide into three parts: exogenous fever, lung-stomach excess heat and internal heat due to yin deficiency. Generally, exogenous fever refers to common cold, but it also can be seen at the onset of acute infectious disease. For young and vulnerable children who are easy to get accompanied symptoms after getting the disease, it should be more cautious to treat them.

Only some acute fever and functional fever originated from viral upper respiratory infection are introduced in this section.

二、病因病机

1. 中医观点

中医认为小儿发热与外感和阴虚有关。

（1）外感发热由于小儿体质偏弱，抗邪能力不足，加之冷热不知调节，家长护理不周，易为风寒外邪所侵，邪气侵袭体表，卫外之阳被郁而致发热。

（2）阴虚内热小儿体质虚弱，先天不足或后天营养失调或久病伤阴而致肺肾不足，阴液亏损引起发热。

2. 西医观点

西医认为引致发热的原因可分为感染性和非感染性两方面。

Ⅱ. Etiology and Pathology

1. Traditional Chinese Medicine Opinion

Traditional Chinese Medicine believes that fever are related with exogenous contraction and yin deficiency.

（1）Exogenous fever: As children are too weak to resist evils and regulate temperature by themselves, along with culpable care by their parents, children can be easily attacked by wind and cold. Evil qi attacks the body surface, and the yang qi which defends the body surface is prevented so that fever is caused.

（2）Internal heat due to yin deficiency: Due to weak physique, poor prenatal essence, acquired malnutrition, chronic illness due to lung and kidney yin deficiency, yin fluid losses and then causes fever.

2. Western Medicine Opinion

Western medicine believes that the cause of fever can be divided into two aspects: infection and non-infection.

三、诊断和鉴别诊断

1. 诊断要点

（1）根据小儿体温升高（肛温高于 37.5 ℃）。

(2)查体：咽部可充血,听诊闻及两肺呼吸音增粗,或干、湿啰音。

(3)实验室检查血常规示白细胞总数增高,中性粒细胞增高。

(4)胸部 X 线检查可发现肺纹理增粗或可见炎症阴影。

2. 鉴别诊断

非感染性与感染性发热的鉴别：感染性发热一般由于病毒或细菌引起,有一定热型,体检时可发现相应的阳性体征。血常规可见白细胞总数增高、中性粒细胞增高、红细胞沉降率加快等。而非感染性发热一般无外界感染源,故两者可鉴别。

Ⅲ. Diagnosis and Differential Diagnosis

1. Essentials of Diagnosis

(1) The rise of children's temperature (Anal temperature is higher than 37.5 ℃).

(2) Physical examination: Pharyngeal is hyperemia, and we can hear wheeze of the two lungs, or rhonchi and moist crackles.

(3) Laboratory examination of blood routine examination showed leukocytosis, neutrophil leukocytosis.

(4) Chest X-ray examination can find thickened lung texture or visible shadow of the inflammation.

2. Differential Diagnosis

Identification of non-infectious and infectious fever: With a certain heat type, infectious fever is usually caused by viruses and bacteria. Physical examination can find the corresponding positive signs. Blood routine examination showed leukocytosis, neutrophil leukocytosis, quick blood sedimentation and so on. Non-infectious fever generally has no external source of infection, so the two can be identified.

四、推拿治疗

1. 辨证分型

(1)外感发热：发热、头痛、怕冷、无汗、鼻塞、流涕、苔薄白、指纹鲜红,为风寒；发热、微汗出、口干、咽痛、鼻流黄涕、苔薄黄、指纹红紫,为风热。

(2)阴虚内热：午后发热,手足心热,形瘦,盗汗,食欲减退,脉细数,舌红苔剥,指纹淡紫。

(3)肺胃实热：高热、面红、气促、不思饮食、便秘烦躁、渴而引饮、舌红苔燥、指纹深紫。

2. 辨证论治

(1)外感发热。

治则：清热解表,发散外邪。

处方：推攒竹、推坎宫、揉太阳、清肺经、清天河水。风寒者加推三关,掐揉二扇门、拿风池;风热者加推脊。

方义:清肺经、清天河水宣肺清热;推攒竹、推坎宫、揉太阳疏风解表,发散外邪;风寒者加推三关,掐揉二扇门、拿风池发汗解表祛散风寒。风热者加推脊、多清天河水以清热解表。

(2)阴虚内热。

治则:滋阴清热。

处方:补脾经、补肺经、揉上马、清天河水、推涌泉,按揉足三里、运内劳宫。

方义:补脾经、揉上马滋肾养肺,滋补阴液,配清天河水、运内劳宫以清虚热;补肺经、按揉足三里健脾和胃,增进饮食;推涌泉引热下行以退虚热。

(3)肺胃实热。

治则:清泻里热,理气消食。

处方:清肺经、清胃经、清大肠、揉板门、运内八卦、清天河水、退六腑、揉天枢。

方义:清肺经、清胃经清肺、胃两经实热,配清大肠、揉天枢疏调肠府积滞以通便泻火;清天河水、退六腑清热除烦;揉板门、运内八卦理气消食。

Ⅳ. Tuina Treatment

1. Syndrome Differentiation

(1) Exogenous fever: wind-cold contraction is characterized by fever, headache, aversion to cold, no sweat, stuffy nose, runny nose, thin white fur, and red superficial venule of the index finger; wind heat contraction is characterized by fever, slight sweating, dry mouth, sore throat, and nasal discharge of yellow snivel, thin and yellow tongue fur, red and purple superficial venule of the index finger.

(2) Internal heat due to yin deficiency: afternoon fever, hot feeling in hand and foot, emaciation, night sweating, loss of appetite, thready pulse, red tongue, and purple superficial venule of the index finger.

(3) Excessive heat in lung and stomach: high fever, red face, shortness of breath, no appetite, constipation, irritability, thirst with desire to drink, dry red tongue, and deep purple superficial venule of the index finger.

2. Treatment Based on Syndrome Differentiation

(1) Exogenous fever

Therapeutic principle: clear heat and diaphoresis

Formula: push Cuanzhu (BL 2), Kangong, Taiyang (EX-HN5), clear the lung meridian and Tianhe water. People who get wind cold should be massaged Sanguan, Ershanmeng, Fengchi (GB 20). People who get wind heat should be massaged spine.

Mechanism of prescription: clear the lung meridian and Tianhe water to disperse lung qi and clear heat. Massage Cuanzhu (BL 2), Kangong, Taiyang (EX-HN5) to treat diaphoresis and disperse wind and evil. For people who get wind cold, massaging Sanguan, Ershanmeng, Fengchi (GB 20) can treat diaphoresis and disperse wind cold. For people who get wind heat, massaging spine and clearing Tianhe water can clear heat and relieve diaphoresis.

(2) Internal heat due to yin deficiency

Therapeutic principle: nourish yin and clear heat.

Formula: Nourish spleen and lung meridian. Massage Shangma, Yongquan, Zu Sanli (ST 36) and Nei laogong (PC 8). Clear Tianhe water.

Mechanism of prescription: nourish spleen meridian and massage Shangma to nourish kidney, lung and yin fluid. Clear Tianhe water and massage Nei laogong (PC 8) to clear deficiency-heat. Nourish lung meridian and massage Zu Sanli (ST 36) to strength spleen and stomach so that we can eat more. Massage Yongquan (KI 1) to lead the heat down to clear deficiency-heat.

(3) Excessive heat in lung and stomach

Therapeutic principle: clear inner heat and regulate the flow of qi to digest food.

Formula: Clear lung, stomach and large intestine meridian. Massage Banmeng, Neibagua, Tianshu (ST 25). Clear Tianhe water and six organs. Knead Tianshu (ST25).

Mechanism of prescription: clear lung and stomach meridians to clear the heat in lung and stomach meridian. Clear large intestine and massage Tianshu (ST 25) to purge fire by defecation. Clear Tianhe water and six organs to clear heat. Massage Banmeng and Neibagua to regulate the flow of qi to digest food.

五、预防与转归

1. 预防

加强护理,慎衣食,适寒热,避风邪,防外感;饮食有节,以免损害脾胃;病后注意营养,以免气血津液亏损;发热高且不退,可一日推拿 2—3 次。

2. 转归

小儿发热需查明原因,针对病因采取相应的治疗措施。若病因明确,措施得当,小儿发热可痊愈。对于年幼体弱的小儿则应注意防止其发热后出现兼证、变证。

Ⅴ. Prevention and Development

1. Prevention

To strengthen nursing, be careful to cloth and food; be suitable to cold and heat; avoid pathogenic wind and exogenous evils; proper diet in case of impairing spleen and stomach; supplement the nutrients after the disease in case of impairing qi-blood-body fluid;

for hyperpyrexia that can't be reduced, we can Tuina twice or three times a day.

2. Development

We need to find out the reason why the children get a fever, and take corresponding measures according to the different etiologies. If the etiology is clear, the measures are correct and the disease can be cured. To the weaker children, we need to avoid accompanying symptoms or deteriorated case after the fever.

第五节   遗   尿
Section Five   Enuresis

一、概念

遗尿是指 3 岁以上的小儿在睡眠中小便自遗、醒后方觉的一种病证,又称尿床、夜尿症。3 岁以下的小儿,由于脑髓未充,智力未健,正常的排尿习惯尚未养成,尿床不属病态。年长小儿因贪玩少睡、精神过度疲劳、睡前多饮等偶尔尿床者,也不必治疗。

本证相当于西医学中大脑皮质、皮质下中枢功能失调引起的遗尿。

Ⅰ. Definition

Enuresis, a disease of involuntary emptying of the urinary bladder during sleep, occurs in children above the age of 3, which is discovered after wakening. It is also known as bedwetting and nocturnal enuresis. Bedwetting is not a morbid condition for children under the age of 3, because they have insufficient brains, unsound intelligence, and they have not developed normal voiding habits yet. Older children occasionally wet the bed for the reasons of much fun and less sleep, mental fatigue, too much bedtime drink and etc. This case needn't to be treated.

This syndrome is equivalent to enuresis in Western medicine which is caused by dysfunction of the cerebral cortex and subcortical central.

二、病因病机

1. 中医观点

中医认为,肾主水、司二便。遗尿的发生主要责之于肾,多由于肾气不足,下元虚寒,致膀胱气化失司,不能制约水道而发生遗尿。此外,肺脾气虚、固摄无权,或肝经郁热、疏泄太过、湿热下注亦可引起遗尿。

2. 西医观点

西医将之分为器质性和功能性两种。小儿遗尿,以小男孩多见,多属功能性,其原因一部分是因功能发育上的不成熟(如膀胱肌肉控制排尿功能差,膀胱容量较小)及睡眠过深不易醒觉等;另一部分由于情绪上的影响,如入学紧张、离开父母。有的孩子以遗尿引起父母的关心,因而遗尿成为心理障碍独特的一种形式。小儿由于患病后身体虚弱,居住环境的改变、白天过度疲劳和兴奋,均可使原先已经控制的排尿功能丧失而出现遗尿。

II. Etiology and Pathology

1. Traditional Chinese Medicine Opinion

Traditional Chinese medicine holds that kidney controls the water, urination and defecation. Enuresis is mainly caused by deficiency of kidney qi and cold-deficiency of lower energizer, resulting in dysfunction of qi transformation of bladder and unregulated waterways. In addition, qi deficiency of lung and spleen leading to the loss of controlling function, as well as heat stagnation in liver meridian and too much catharsis can cause enuresis.

2. Western Medicine Opinion

Western medicine divides enuresis into organic ones and functional ones. Pediatric Enuresis, more common in little boys, is mostly functional enuresis. And part of the reason is the immaturity functional development (eg. Cystatin muscle's urination controlling function is poor and bladder capacity is small.), deep sleep and difficulty to wake up. Another part of the reason is the influence of emotional stress, such as going to school and leaving their parents. Some children make enuresis as a method to obtain parental care, thus it becomes a unique form of psychological disorder. The urination controlling function can be lost and lead to enuresis because of the weakness after illness, the change of living environment, daytime fatigue and excitement.

三、诊断和鉴别诊断

1. 诊断要点

(1) 发病年龄在 3 周岁以上。

(2) 睡眠较深,不易唤醒,每夜或隔天发生尿床,甚则每夜遗尿 1—2 次以上者。

(3) 尿常规及尿培养无异常发现。

(4) X 线检查,部分患儿可发现隐性脊柱裂,或做泌尿道造影可见畸形。

2. 鉴别诊断

尿崩症:患儿有多饮、多尿病史,尿比重多为 1.001—1.000。禁水试验示尿比重升高不明显、尿量不减,体重及血压下降。

III. Diagnosis and Differential Diagnosis

1. Essentials of Diagnosis

(1) The disease attacks children more than 3 years old.

(2) The children are in deep sleep and are difficult to be wakened up. Enuresis occurs every night or every two days, even more then 1 or 2 times in one night.

(3) No abnormal findings are present in routine urine test and urine culture.

(4) Some patients may find hidden spina bifida in X-ray examination or urinary tract malformations in urinary tract angiography.

2. Differential Diagnosis

Diabetes insipidus: children have a history of more drinking and more urine, with specific gravity of urine between 1. 001 and 1. 000. Water-deprivation test shows no obvious promotion in urine specific gravity, no reduction in urination, weight and blood pressure.

四、推拿治疗

1. 辨证分型

(1) 肾气不足：睡眠中不自主排尿，如白天疲劳，天气阴雨时更易发生，轻则数夜遗尿一次，重则每夜遗尿一至二次，甚或更多。遗尿病久可见患儿面色㿠白、智力减退、精神不振、头晕腰酸、四肢不温等症，舌淡、脉沉细。

(2) 肝经湿热：睡中遗尿、尿量不多、色黄腥臊、夜梦纷纭、急躁易怒、面赤唇红、口干、舌红、苔黄、脉多弦数。

2. 辨证施治

(1) 肾气不足。

治则：温补脾神，固涩下元。

处方：补脾经、补肺经、补肾经、推三关、揉外劳、按揉百会、揉丹田、按揉肾俞、擦腰骶部、按揉三阴交。

方义：揉丹田、按揉肾俞、擦腰骶部、补肾经以温补肾气，壮命门之火，固涩下元；补脾经、补肺经、推三关健脾益气，补肺脾气血；揉外劳、按揉百会温阳升提；按揉三阴交以通调水道。

(2) 肝经湿热。

治则：疏肝解郁，清热利湿。

处方：清肝经、清小肠、退六腑、揉丹田、揉肾经、揉龟尾、按揉三阴交。

方义：清肝经、清小肠、退六腑能疏肝解郁，清热、利小便；揉丹田、揉肾经、揉龟尾可补益肾气，固涩下元；三阴交为足三阴经的交会穴，按揉三阴交能调理肝肾。

Ⅳ. Tuina treatment

1. Syndrome Differentiation

(1) Deficiency of kidney qi: Involuntary urination during sleep especially when the children are tired in day or weather is rainy. In mild cases, it occurs once in

several nights, while in severe cases, the kid urinates several times in a night. In a long term, there are symptoms like pale complexion, mental retardation, poor spirit, dizziness and lumbar soreness, cold limbs, light-colored tongue and deep-thin pulse.

(2) Damp-heat in liver meridian: Involuntary urination during sleep, scanty, yellow and smelly urine, dreaminess, anxiety and irritation, red complexion and lips, dry mouth, red tongue with yellow coating and fast-tight pulse.

2. Treatment Based on Syndrome Differentiation

(1) Deficiency of kidney qi

Therapeutic principle: Warm the spirit of spleen and firm the spirit of kidney.

Formula: Supplement the spleen meridian, the lung meridian and the kidney meridian. Rub Sanguan, press Wailao, Baihui (GV 20), Dantian, Shenshu (BL 23), Sanyin Jiao (SP 6) and lumbosacral portion.

Mechanism of prescription: Press Dantian, Shenshu (BL 23) and lumbosacral portion in order to warm and supplement kidney qi, promote the fire in Mingmen and firm the spirit of kidney. Rub Sanguan in order to supplement the spleen meridian and the lung meridian and promote the qi and blood of lung and spleen. Press Wailao and Baihui (GV 20) to warm and elevate yang qi. Press Sanyin Jiao (SP 6) to mediate channels.

(2) Damp-heat in liver meridian

Therapeutic principle: Sooth liver, clear the heat and moisten liver meridian.

Formula: Clear liver meridian, small intestine and Fu organs. Press Dantian, Guiwei, Sanyin Jiao (SP 6) and kidney meridian.

Mechanism of prescription: Clear liver meridian, small intestine and Fu organs in order to sooth the liver, clear heat and promote urine. Knead Dantian, Guiwei and kidney meridian to promote Kidney qi and firm the spirit of kidney. Sanyin Jiao (SP 6) is the rendezvous point of three yin meridians of feet and pressing it can regulate liver and kidney.

五、预防与转归

1. 预防

注意培养按时排尿的习惯。睡前不给饮水和其他流质。白天不使其过度疲劳;睡前不使其过度兴奋;睡中应按其平素遗尿时间,提前唤醒,让其小便。对患儿应注意耐心教导,以免增加精神负担,以致影响身心健康。

2. 转归

小儿遗尿及早治疗则疗效较好,若治疗失时,病迁日久,就会影响儿童的身心健康。

Ⅴ. Prevention and Development

1. Prevention

Develop a habit of urination on time. Don't drink water or other liquid before sleep. Do not be excessively tired at day or excessively excited at night. Patients should wake up the children to urinate according to their usual time of urination. Be patient to the children so that they won't be under pressure and be affected physically and psychologically.

2. Development

Involuntary urination of children can achieve better curative effect in early treatment. If the treatment is not in time or the disease prolongs, involuntary urination will have bad effects on children physically and psychologically.

第六节 夜 啼
Section Six Night Crying

一、概念

夜啼是指小儿经常在夜间啼哭不眠,甚至通宵达旦。白天如常,入夜则啼哭,或每夜定时啼哭者称"夜啼"。民间俗称"哭啼郎"。有时阵阵啼哭,哭后仍能入睡。本病多见于半岁以内的婴幼儿。

本证与西医学的小儿睡眠障碍中的夜惊等相近。

Ⅰ. Definition

Night crying refers to an infant often crying and being restless at night or even keeping crying throughout the night. The infant may be normal in daytime but cry at night or at a certain time every night. It's commonly known as "crying boy" (Kuti Lang). Sometimes after crying, the kid can fall asleep. The disease is more common in infants less than six months.

This syndrome is similar to the pediatric sleep disorders due to the night terrors in Western medicine.

二、病因病机

1. 中医观点

中医认为夜啼的发生与脾寒、心热、惊骇、食积有关。

（1）脾寒：婴儿素禀虚弱，脾常不足，至夜阴盛，脾为阴中之阴，若护理略有失意，寒邪内侵，脾寒乃生。夜属阴，阴胜脾寒愈盛，寒邪凝滞，气机不通，故入夜腹痛而啼。

（2）心热：乳母平日恣食辛辣肥甘，或焦躁炙搏动火之食物，或贪服性热之药，火伏热郁，积热上炎。心主火属阳，阳为人生之正气，至夜则阴盛而阳衰，阳衰则无力与邪热相搏，正不胜邪，则邪热乘心，心属火恶热而致夜间烦躁啼哭。

（3）惊骇：小儿神气不足，心气怯弱，如有目触异物，耳闻异声，使心神不宁，神志不安，常在梦中哭而作惊，故在夜间惊啼不寐。

（4）食积：婴儿乳食不节，内伤脾胃，胃不和则卧不安，因脾胃运化失司，乳食积滞，入夜而啼。

2. 西医观点

西医认为小儿夜啼的原因尚不清楚。一般追问病史，常可发现患儿白天生活睡眠制度不规则或护理不当，如白天或睡前游嬉过度、兴奋紧张，或夜间不能按时睡眠，或睡觉时衣被过厚等。

Ⅱ. Etiology and Pathology

1. Traditional Chinese Medicine Opinion

It is believed in traditional Chinese medicine that night crying is related to spleen-cold, heart-hot, terror and indigestion.

(1) Spleen-cold: The infant is congenitally weak with insufficient spleen. The yin becomes excessive at night and the spleen is yin within yin. If nursing is improper, pathogenic cold will invade so that the spleen-cold is born. Since the night belongs to yin, the more excessive yin is, the more spleen-cold will be born. As the pathogenic cold stagnate, the qi will be blocked. Thus the infant cries at night due to the abdominal pain.

(2) Heart-heat: The nursing mother usually eats the greasy and spicy food, or fried and burned food, or prefers the hot-natured drugs, so the pathogenic fire and heat stagnate and accumulated heat flames up. Heart governs the fire and belongs to yang which is the healthy qi of the human body. When the night comes, yin becomes excessive and yang becomes deficient for which it's weak to fight against evil heat so that vital qi can't conquer the evil qi. The pathogenic heat can trouble heart that belongs to yang and intolerant to heat, making the infant uncomfortable and crying incessantly.

(3) Terror: The infant is weak in spirit-qi and deficient in heart-qi. If he sees something strange or hears something abnormal, the uneasiness and restless will make the infant cry with fear during dreams, resulting in crying with fear and insomnia at night.

(4) Indigestion: The infant eats and drinks food and milk without temperance, so the spleen and stomach are damaged and disordered stomach leads to insomnia with restlessness. Thus the infant cries at night due to the stagnation of milk and food caused by the failure of the transporting and transforming function of the spleen and stomach.

2. Western Medicine Opinion

The reason of infant night crying is still unknown in western medicine. Further questions about the patient's history may help to find the manifestations like irregular sleep and activities at daytime, improper care such as too much playing at daytime or before sleep or excitement, inability to sleep at time or wearing too thick clothes or quilt when sleeping.

三、诊断和鉴别诊断

1. 诊断要点

（1）根据患儿夜间无明显诱因而哭闹不止,查体无明显体征,并排除小儿发热、佝偻病、饶虫病、骨和关节结核等病证引起的夜间哭闹。

（2）患儿精神状态良好,无发绀,呼吸正常,体温正常,全腹平软。

2. 鉴别诊断

遗尿:夜啼患儿常在夜间无明显诱因而哭闹不止,而遗尿是指 3 岁以上的小儿在睡眠中不知不觉地将小便尿在床上而引起的啼哭,故不难鉴别。

Ⅲ. Diagnosis and Differential Diagnosis

1. Essentials of Diagnosis

（1）It can be diagnosed according to the children crying at night without obvious incentive or signs in physical examination. Those caused by fever, rickets, enterobiasis, tuberculosis of bones and joints and other diseases need to be ruled out.

（2）Children show good mental state, no cyanosis, normal breathing, normal body temperature, flat and soft abdomen.

2. Differential Diagnosis

Enuresis: The children with night crying often cry at night without obvious incentive while enuresis refers to children over 3 years old crying due to peeing in the bed unconsciously during sleep. It's easy to make a differential diagnosis.

四、推拿治疗

1. 辨证分型

（1）脾脏虚寒:睡喜伏卧,曲腰而啼,四肢欠温,食少便溏,面色青白,唇舌淡白,舌苔薄白,脉象沉细,指纹青红。

（2）心经积热：睡喜仰卧,见灯火则啼哭愈甚,烦躁不安,小便短赤,或大便秘结,面赤唇红,舌尖红,舌苔白,脉数有力,指纹青紫。

（3）惊骇恐惧：睡中时作惊惕,唇与面色乍青乍白,紧偎母怀,脉、舌多无异常变化,或夜间脉来弦数。

（4）乳食积滞：夜间阵发啼哭,脘腹胀满,呕吐乳块,大便酸臭,舌苔厚,指纹紫。

2. 辨证施治

（1）脾脏虚寒。

治则：温中健脾。

处方：补脾经、推三关、摩腹、揉中脘。

方义：补脾经、摩腹、揉中脘穴以温中健脾,推三关以温全身之阳。

（2）心经积热。

治则：清心导赤。

处方：清心经、清小肠、清天河水、揉总筋、揉内劳宫。

方义：清心经、清天河水以清热退心火;清小肠以导赤而泻心火;揉总筋、揉内劳宫以清心经热。

（3）惊骇恐惧。

治则：镇惊安神。

处方：推攒竹、清肝经、揉小天心、揉五指节。

方义：推攒竹、清肝经、揉小天心以镇惊除烦;揉五指节以安神。

（4）乳食积滞。

治则：消食导滞。

处方：清补脾经(先清后不补)、清大肠、摩腹、揉中脘、揉天枢、揉脐、推下七节。

方义：清补脾经以健脾利湿;清大肠、推下七节以清利肠府,泻热通便;摩腹、揉中脘、揉天枢、揉脐以健脾和胃消食导滞。

Ⅳ. Tuina Treatment

1. Syndrome Differentiation

（1）Deficiency-cold of spleen: preference to sleeping on the chest; crying with waist curved; cold limbs; small intake of food and diarrhea; blue and white complexion; pale lips and tongue; thin and white coating with sink and fine pulse; blue and red superficial venule of the index finger.

（2）Heat accumulating in the heart meridian: preference to sleeping on the back; crying more fiercely when he sees light and fire; vexation and restlessness; short and red urine or constipation; red face and lips; red tip of the tongue; white tongue coating; rapid and forceful pulse; blue and purple superficial venule of the index finger.

(3) Fright and terror: The infant sometimes gets frightened and restless at sleep; face and lips turn to blue and the next time to white; closely hugging mother; normal pulse and tongue, or string and rapid pulse at night.

(4) Indigestion of milk and food: nocturnal paroxysmal crying; abdominal distension; vomiting the curdling of the milk; sour-smelling malodorous stool; thick tongue coating; purple superficial venule of the index finger.

2. Treatment Based on Syndrome Differentiation

(1) Deficiency-cold of Spleen

Therapeutic principle: warm the middle and invigorate the spleen.

Formula: nourish Pijing, push Sanguan, rub abdomen, knead Zhongwan (CV 12).

Mechanism of prescription: to warm the middle and invigorate the spleen by nourishing Pijing, rubbing abdomen, kneading Zhongwan (CV 12) and to warm the yang qi of the whole body by pushing Sanguan.

(2) Heat accumulating in the heart meridian

Therapeutic principle: clear heart by purging reddish urine.

Formula: clear heart meridian, small intestine and Tianhe water, knead Zongjin and Neilaogong (PC 8).

Mechanism of prescription: clearing heart meridian and Tianhe water can fail heart fire; clearing small intestine can purge heart fire; kneading Zongjin and Nei Laogong (PC 8) to clear heart meridian heat.

(3) Fright and terror

Therapeutic principle: tranquilize and quiet mind.

Formula: push Cuanzhu (BL 2), clear liver meridian, knead Xiaotianxin and Wuzhijie.

Mechanism of prescription: pushing Cuanzhu(BL 2), clearing liver meridian and kneading Xiaotianxin can tranquilize, while kneading Wuzhijie can quiet mind.

(4) Indigestion of milk and food

Therapeutic principle: promote digestion and remove stagnation.

Formula: clear and nourish spleen meridian (clearing first but not followed with nourishing); rub abdomen; knead Zhongwan (CV 12), Tianshu (ST 25) and umbilicus; push Xiaqijie.

Mechanism of prescription: clearing and nourishing spleen meridian to invigorate spleen; clearing large intestine and pushing Xiaqijie can clear intestine to purge heat to relax bowels; kneading Zhongwan (CV 12), Tianshu (ST 25) and umbilicus can invigorate spleen and stomach, promote digestion and resolve stagnation.

五、预防与转归

1. 预防

平素寒温宜调护,防受寒受凉;饮食不宜过凉。新生儿当服黄连汤少许,以解胎热;生后不宜多服香燥炙煿之品。小儿气弱,避免异声异物,防惊恐。饮食有节,防过饱伤脾。晚间啼哭的原因甚多,去除原因,则其哭自止。

2. 转归

小儿夜啼一般易治,调治得当,则数日可愈,若调治失宜,则迁延数月,严重者可对小儿身心健康产生影响。

Ⅴ. Prevention and Development

1. Prevention

Keep warm; diet should not be too cold. Newborn baby should drink a bit of Coptidis Decoction to resolve fetal heat. Don't use too much drugs which is dry and aromatic. For babies who are weak of qi, avoid abnormal sounds and abnormal objects to prevent panic. Have a proper diet to prevent spleen impairment caused by excessive intake. There are many reasons for night crying. Once the reasons are removed, the crying will stop.

2. Development

It is usually easy to cure nocturnal crying in infants. It takes a few days to cure the disease when it was treated correctly. But it could also last for several months by improper treatment, or even cause damage physically and psychologically.

第三部分
针灸和其他
Part Three Acupuncture and
Moxibustion and the Others

针灸疗法是祖国医学的一部分,千百年来,对保卫健康,抵御疾病,有过卓越的贡献,为广大群众所信赖。它包括针刺、灸法、刮痧、拔罐四大部分。它是一种通过经络、腧穴的传导作用,以及应用一定的操作法,来治疗全身疾病的"内病外治"的医术。

As a part of Chinese medicine, acupuncture and moxibustion have made great contributions to keeping health and warding diseases and have been trusted by our people. It includes four parts, namely, acupuncture, moxibustion, skin scraping and cupping therapy. By using the transmitting functions of meridians and acupoints, these four parts can treat diseases of the whole body externally with some operational techniques.

第十章 针刺技术
Chapter Ten Acupuncture

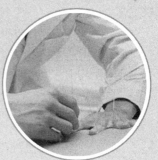

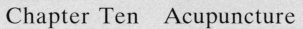

一、概念

针刺是指在中医理论的指导下,采用不同针具,刺激人体的一定部位(经络腧穴),并运用各种手法以调整阴阳、防治疾病的方法。

Ⅰ. Definition

Under the guidance of traditional Chinese medicine (TCM), acupuncture is one of the therapeutic methods by means of needling with certain manipulation to stimulate certain part (meridians and acupoints) to adjust yin and yang, prevent and treat diseases.

二、治疗原理

经络腧穴理论是针刺疗法的基本理论。经络是人体运行气血、协调阴阳、联络脏腑、沟通内外、贯串上下的通路。针刺治疗疾病就是通过激发经气的调整功能,来调节脏腑的功能状态。

Ⅱ. Rationale of Treatment

The theory of meridians and acupoints is the basic theory of acupuncture therapy. Meridians refer to the routes that transport qi and blood, regulate yin and yang, connect the zang-organs and fu-organs, associate the external with the internal as well as the upper with the lower. The basic theory of acupuncture in treating diseases lies in their regulating functions through activating meridian qi to adjust the states of the viscera.

三、分类

按照针刺部位的不同,临床上常见三种不同的类型：针治部位以身体各处为主,称为"体针";仅取耳穴治疗疾病,称为"耳针";刺激区域集中在头部,称为"头皮针"。

Ⅲ. Classification

According to the different locations of the needling, there are three common classifications: body acupuncture which means to needle the acupoints mainly located on the body; ear acupuncture that refers to needling the acupoints mainly located on the ear; scalp acupuncture which means to puncture the acupoints mainly located on the scalp.

四、适应证

针刺疗法具有适应证广、疗效明显、操作方便、经济安全等优点。常见的适应证有腰痛、落枕、周围性面神经炎、失眠、泄泻、月经不调、带状疱疹等。

Ⅳ. Indications

Acupuncture has many advantages, such as wide indications, obvious effects, convenient operation, low cost with safety. Common indications are low back pain, stiff neck, peripheral facial paralysis, insomnia, diarrhea, irregular menstruation, herpes zoster.

五、禁忌证

(1) 患者在过度饥饿、暴饮暴食、醉酒后及精神过度紧张时,禁止针刺。
(2) 孕妇的少腹部、腰骶部、会阴部禁止针刺。
(3) 严重的过敏性、感染性皮肤病者,以及患有出血性疾病的患者禁止针刺。
(4) 小儿囟门未闭时头顶部禁止针刺。

Ⅴ. Contraindication

(1) It is forbidden to give acupuncture treatment to those who are starving, crapulent, drunk or very nervous.
(2) The lower abdomen, lumbosacral, and perineum of the pregnant women are

forbidden to be needled.

（3）Patients with severe infection, contagious skin diseases and ulcer, and hemorrhagic tendency should not be needled.

（4）Acupoints on the vertex of infants should not be needled when the fontanel is not closed.

第二节　技术操作
Section Two　Operation Techniques

一、器械材料准备

针具选择应以具有一定的硬度、弹性和韧性。临床应用一般以不锈钢为多,粗细为0.32—0.38 mm 和长短为 25—75 mm 的毫针最为常用。根据病人的性别、年龄的长幼、形体的肥瘦、体质的强弱.病情的虚实、病变部位的表里浅深和所取腧穴所在的具体部位,选择长短、粗细适宜的针具。如男性、体壮、形肥,且病变部位较深者,可选稍粗稍长的毫针。反之若女性、体弱、形瘦,而病变部位较浅者,就应选用较短、较细的针具。至于根据腧穴的所在具体部位进行选针,一般是皮薄肉少之处和针刺较浅的腧穴,选针宜短而针身宜细;皮厚肉多而针刺宜深的腧穴宜选用针身稍长、稍粗的毫针。

Ⅰ. Materials

Needles with a certain degree of hardness, elasticity and toughness should be selected. Most of them are made of stainless steel, 0.32 - 0.38 mm in diameter and 25 - 75 mm in length. Proper needles are selected based on the patient's gender, age, figure, constitution, location of acupoints. Slightly longer and thicker needle should be selected for the male, the strong, the fat and those with deeper lesions. In contrast, a shorter, thinner needle should be used for women, the weak, the thin and those with shallow lesions. As to the acupoints location, the area with thin skin and less muscles or acupoints that need to be needled shallowly should be punctured by short and thin needles; the area with thick skin and strong muscles or acupoints that need to be needled deeply deep should be punctured by longer and thicker needles.

二、患者选择合适的体位

针刺时必须要求病人采取和保持一定的体位姿势,以便于取穴、保持留针、防止针身弯曲折断和晕针。针前嘱咐病人尽量把身体姿势放得舒服自然,能坚持较长时间而不移动。临床上针刺时常用的体位,有如下几种:

（1）仰卧位:适宜于取头、面、胸、腹部腧穴,和上、下肢部分腧穴。

（2）侧卧位：适宜于取身体侧面腧穴和上、下肢的部分腧穴。

（3）俯卧位：适宜于取头、项、脊背、腰骶部腧穴，和下肢背侧及上肢部分腧穴。

（4）仰靠坐位：适宜于取前头、颜面和颈前等部位的腧穴。

（5）俯伏坐位：适宜于取后头和项、背部的腧穴。

（6）侧伏坐位：适宜于取头部的一侧，面颊及耳前后部位的腧穴。

Ⅱ. Choose the Appropriate Posture

Appropriate posture of the patient is important for correct location of acupoints, prolonged retention of the needle and prevention of bending and breaking the needle as well as fainting during treatment. Before needling, ask the patient to relax himself, keep a comfortable and natural posture so as to maintain the position for a longer time. The following are some of the commonly selected postures:

（1）Supine: suitable for the acupoints on the head, face, chest, abdominal regions and the limbs.

（2）Lateral recumbent posture: suitable for the acupoints on the posterior of the head, neck, back and the lateral side of the limbs.

（3）Prone: suitable for the acupoints on the posterior of the head, neck, back lumbar and buttock regions, and the posterior side of the limbs.

（4）Sitting in supine: suitable for the acupoints on the head, face as well as the upper chest region.

（5）Sitting in prone: suitable for the acupoints on the posterior of the head, neck, and back.

（6）Sitting with inclining position: suitable for the acupoints on the lateral side of the head and ear area.

三、定穴

针刺前医者必须将施术的腧穴定位准确，简称"定穴"。医者以手指在穴位处进行揣、摸、按、循，找出具有指感的穴位称为"揣穴"。

Ⅲ. Locating Acupoints

Locating acupoints: The acupoints should be located accurately. Searching acupoints: the acupuncturist presses and rubs around the acupoint to decide its exact location.

四、消毒

针刺前必须做好消毒工作，其中包括腧穴部位和医者手指的消毒。

方法如下：在需要针刺的腧穴部位消毒时，可用 75% 酒精棉球拭擦即可。在拭擦时应由腧穴部位的中心向四周绕圈擦拭。或先用 25% 碘酒棉球拭擦，然后再用 75% 酒精棉球涂擦消毒。当腧穴消毒后，切忌接触污物，以免重新污染。

医者手指的消毒：在施术前，医者应先用肥皂水将手洗刷干净，待干后再用 75% 酒精棉球擦拭即可。施术时医者应尽量避免手指直接接触针体，如必须接触针体时，可用消毒干棉球作间隔物，以保持针身无菌。

Ⅳ. Sterilization

Sterilization includes the sterilization of the needling region, and the hands of acupuncturist.

The area selected for needling must be sterilized with a 75% alcohol cotton ball or with 25% iodine first and then with a 75% alcohol cotton ball. The selected area is sterilized from the center to the sides. After sterilization, recontamination should be avoided.

Before needling, the acupuncturist should wash his hands with soup, and then sterilize the hands with 75% alcohol cotton balls. During needling, avoid contacting the needle directly. If necessary, use a sterilized cotton ball to keep the needle uncontaminated.

五、进针

在进行针刺操作时，一般应双手协同操作，紧密配合。左手爪切按压所刺部位或辅助针身，故称左手为"押手"；右手持针操作，主要是以拇、食、中三指挟持针柄，其状如持毛笔，故右手称为"刺手"。

1. 爪切法

又称指切法。以左手拇指或食指之指甲掐切穴位上，右手持针将针紧靠左手指甲缘刺入皮下的手法。

2. 夹持进针法

夹持进针法是指用左手拇、食二指持捏消毒干棉球，夹住针身下端，将针尖固定在所刺腧穴的皮肤表面位置；右手捻动针柄，将针刺入腧穴。此法适用于长针进针。

3. 舒张进针法

舒张进针法是指用左手拇、食二指将所刺腧穴部位的皮肤向两侧撑开，使皮肤绷紧；右手持针，使针从左手拇、食二指的中间刺入。此法主要用于皮肤松弛部位腧穴。

4. 提捏进针法

指用左手拇、食二指将针刺腧穴部位的皮肤捏起，右手持针，从捏起的上端将针刺入。此法主要用于皮肉浅薄部位的腧穴进针，如印堂穴等。

Ⅴ. Insertion

During needling, two hands should generally cooperate closely with each other. The right hand, known as "puncturing hand", holds needle with the thumb, index finger and middle finger. The left hand, known as "pressing hand", pushes firmly against the area close to the acupoint or presses the needle body from both sides to assist right hand.

1. Nailing Insertion of the Needle

Press the area beside the acupoint with the nail of the thumb or the index finger of left hand; hold the needle with right hand and keep the needle tip closely against the nail, and then insert the needle into the acupoint.

2. Holding Inserting of the Needle

Hold the needle tip with sterilized dry cotton balls held by thumb and index finger of left hand; keep the needle tip on the skin and insert the needle by right hand twirling. This method is suitable for long needles.

3. Relaxed Inserting of the Needle

Stretch the skin where the acupoint is located with the thumb and index finger of the left hand, hold the needle with the right hand and then insert it into the area between the two fingers. This method is suitable for the regions with loose skin.

4. Lifting and Pinching of the Needle

Pinch the skin up around the acupoint with the thumb and index finger of the left hand; insert the needle into the acupoint with right hand. This method is suitable for the acupoints where the muscles are thin like Yintang (EX-HN 3).

六、行针

毫针进针后,为了使患者产生针刺感应,或进一步调整针感的强弱,以及使针感向某一方向扩散、传导而采取的操作方法,称为"行针"。常用的行针手法有提插法和捻转法。

1. 提插法

即将针刺入腧穴一定深度后,施以上提下插动作的操作手法。

2. 捻转法

即将针刺入腧穴一定深度后,施以向前向后捻转动作的操作手法。

Ⅵ. Manipulation

After needling, several methods can be used for inducing needling effect, or adjusting the strength and spreading needling effects. Basic manipulation techniques are twirling-rotating and lifting-thrusting.

1. Twirling-rotating

After the needle is inserted to the desired depth, the needle is twirled and rotated backward and forward with the thumb, index finger and middle finger of right hand.

2. Lifting-thrusting

After the needle is inserted to a certain depth, the needle is lifted and thrusted perpendicularly and continuously.

七、留针

将针刺入腧穴行针施术后，使针留置穴内，称为留针。一般病证只要针下得气而施以适当的补泻手法后，即可出针或留针 10—20 分钟；但对一些特殊病证，如急性腹痛、破伤风、角弓反张、顽固性疼痛或痉挛性病证，即可适当延长留针时间，有时留针可达数小时，以便在留针过程中作间歇性行针，以增强、巩固疗效。

Ⅶ. Retention

Retention means to hold the needle in the acupoint after the manipulation. For common disease, the needles can be withdrawn or be retained for 10 – 20 minutes after the manipulation. But for some special diseases, such as acute abdominal pain, tetanus, opisthotonos, intractable pain or venereal spasm syndrome, the time for retention may be prolonged, sometimes to several hours. At the same time, manipulation can be performed at intervals in order to improve the therapeutic effects.

八、出针

出针时一般先以左手拇、食指按住针孔周围皮肤，右手持针作轻微捻转，慢慢将针提至皮下，然后将针起出，用消毒干棉球揉按针孔，以防出血。若用除疾，开阖补泻时，则应按各自的具体操作要求，将针起出。出针后病人应休息片刻方可活动，医者应检查针数以防遗漏。

Ⅷ. Withdrawal

For the withdrawal of the needle, press the skin around the acupoint slightly with sterilized cotton ball held by left hand, rotate the needle handle gently and lift it slowly to subcutaneous level with the right hand, then withdraw it quickly and press the acupoint with cotton balls to prevent bleeding. If to remove diseases, the doctor needs to operate according to the specific requirements of opening-closing reinforcement and reduction. After the withdrawal, patients should rest for a while before getting up, and the acupuncturist should count the number of the needles to make sure that all the needles are withdrawn.

九、治疗时间及疗程

1. 治疗时间

一般病证针刺治疗时间在 20—30 分钟为宜。

2. 疗程

多数疾病,如面瘫、风湿痹痛等,以针灸 10 次为一疗程。部分急性病证,例如落枕、牙痛,以 3—5 次为一疗程。少数慢性病,疑难病,如肥胖症、中风后遗症,至少一个月为一个疗程。

Ⅸ. Duration and Course of Treatment

1. Duration

Twenty to thirty minutes will be fine for common diseases.

2. Course

Many diseases, such as facial paralysis and arthritis, will need 10 times acupuncture for one course. Some acute diseases, like stiff neck, toothache, will need 3 - 5 times for one course. Some chronic diseases, like obesity, stroke, will take one month for one course.

十、关键技术环节

定穴和揣穴是确定腧穴正确位置,利于进针的准备工作,腧穴的定位正确与否,直接关系到针刺的疗效。

Ⅹ. Key Techniques

Locating acupoints and searching acupoints are prerequisite to the treatment of acupuncture. It is directly closed with the effects of acupuncture.

十一、注意事项

(1) 对精神过度紧张,过于疲劳者,不宜立即针刺。

(2) 孕妇、妇女月经期不宜针刺;小孩囟门未合时,头顶部不宜针刺;皮肤感染、溃疡、瘢痕及肿瘤部位,不宜针刺;凝血功能障碍,有出血倾向者,不宜针刺。

(3) 眼区、颈项部、靠近重要脏器和大血管处的腧穴慎刺。

(4) 针刺手法的轻重应以病人的耐受度为准。对体质虚弱,精神过度紧张者手法宜轻柔。

Ⅺ. Notes

(1) Delay acupuncture treatment to the patient who are very nervous, or over

tired.

（2）Pregnant women and women with menstruation are not suitable for acupuncture. Acupoints on the vertex of infants should not be needled when the fontanel is not closed. Acupoints on the areas with infection, ulcer, scar or tumor should not be needled. Patients with disturbance of blood coagulation and hemorrhagic tendency should not be needled.

（3）Acupoints on the ocular area, neck, or close to the vital organs or large blood vessels should be carefully needled.

（4）The needling methods should be selected according to the tolerance of patients. For those who are very nervous and weak, mild manipulation can be used.

十二、可能的意外情况及处理方案

在针刺治疗过程中,由于患者心理准备不足等多种原因,可能出现如下异常情况,应及时处理。

1. 晕针

由于患者精神过度紧张,体质虚弱,过度疲劳,体位不当或者针刺手法过重等原因,患者在针刺或留针过程中突然出现头晕、恶心、心慌,面色苍白,出冷汗等表现,此时应立即停止针刺,起出全部留针,同时安慰病人,令其平卧,闭目休息,并饮少量温开水,周围环境应避免嘈杂。若症状较重,则可针刺素髎、内关、水沟等穴,促其恢复。如仍不省人事,应采取其他急救措施。

2. 滞针

在针刺行针及起针时,术者手上对在穴位内的针体有涩滞、牵拉、包裹的感觉称滞针。滞针使针体不易被提插、捻转,不易起针。滞针的主要原因是针刺手法不当,使患者的针刺处发生肌肉强直性收缩,致肌纤维缠裹在针体上。应令患者全身放松,并用手按摩针刺部位,使局部肌肉松弛。然后,轻缓向初时行针相反方向捻转,提动针体,缓慢将针起出。

XII. Possible Accidents and Management

In the process of acupuncture treatment, due to lack of psychological preparation of patients and other reasons, it may appear unusual circumstances as follows, which should be taken care in time.

1. Fainting

This is caused by nervousness, delicate constitution, fatigue, improper posture or forceful manipulation. During acupuncture treatment, once the symptoms like dizziness, vertigo, pallor, palpitation, chest distress, nausea, vomiting and cold limbs occur, all the needles should be withdrawn immediately. The acupuncturist should soothe the patient, help him/her lie down and offer some warm water. The patient should be recovered after a short rest. In severe cases, acupoints like Suliao (GV25), Neiguan (PC 6), Shuigou (GV26) can be needled to resuscitate the patient. If the patent stays unconscious, other emergency measures should be taken.

2. Stuck Needle

It refers to the condition that the acupuncturist feels tense and unsmooth beneath the needle and difficult to twirl, rotate, lift and thrust the needle during the manipulation or withdrawn needle. The reason for stuck needle is inappropriate way of manipulation, the nervousness and excessive contraction of local muscle. The acupuncturist should sooth the patient first, massage the local region gently to relax the muscle, and then rotate the needle to the opposite direction with slightly lifting the needle out.

第十一章 灸法技术
Chapter Eleven　Moxibustion

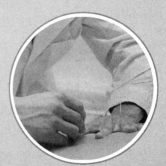

第一节　概　述
Section One　General Introduction

一、概念

灸法，是利用灸火刺激人体经络穴位以防治疾病的一种方法，是针灸疗法的重要组成部分。

Ⅰ. Definition

Moxibustion is a therapy used to treat and prevent diseases by applying burning moxa to stimulate the human body (meridians and acupoints). It is an important part of acupuncture and moxibustion.

二、治疗原理

灸法是用艾绒或其他药物放置在体表的穴位上烧灼、烫熨，借灸火的温和热力以及药物的作用，通过经络的传导，起到温通气血，扶正祛邪，达到治疗疾病和预防保健目的的一种外治方法。

Ⅱ. Rationale of Treatment

Moxibustion is an exterior therapeutic way used to treat and prevent diseases by placing moxa or other drugs on the acupoint on the surface. With burning and ironing, the moderate heat of the moxa and drugs can warm the qi and blood, eliminate pathogenic factors and support healthy qi through the meridians.

三、分类

1. 艾柱灸

将艾绒制成圆锥形的艾团,称为艾柱。治疗时将艾柱置于所灸部位,根据艾柱与皮肤之间是否放置间隔物,又可分为直接灸和间接灸。

2. 直接灸

艾柱直接放在皮肤上施灸。根据灸火烧灼皮肤程度的不同,又分为无瘢痕灸和瘢痕灸。

3. 隔物灸

施灸时在艾柱与皮肤之间放置某种物品,常用生姜、蒜等,以防止烫伤皮肤。

4. 艾条灸

艾条由纸包裹艾绒卷制而成,一般为直径 1.5 厘米,长 20 厘米的圆筒形。

5. 温针灸

将针刺与艾灸合并使用的方法。

Ⅲ. Classification

1. Moxibustion with Moxa Cone

Moxa cone is cone-shaped mugwort wool. It is placed on the acupoint selected for moxibustion. It is either direct or indirect, depending on whether there is something between the moxa cone and the skin.

2. Direct Moxibustion

The moxa is placed directly on the acupoint and ignited. It is either scarring or non-scarring according to the degree of burning over the skin.

3. Stuff-isolation Moxibustion

The moxa cone is isolated from the skin by some materials, such as ginger, garlic, in order to avoid burning the skin.

4. Moxibustion with Moxa Roll

Moxa roll is prepared by wrapping mugwort wool with a piece of paper. It is cylinder shaped 1.5cm in diameter and 20cm in length.

5. Moxibustion with Warmed Needles

It is a method combined with acupuncture and moxibustion.

四、适应证

各类虚寒病证,风寒湿痹痛,寒性腹痛腹泻,哮喘,肺痨等慢性疾病。

Ⅳ. Indications

Deficiency-cold syndrome, arthralgia due to pathogenic wind-cold, abdominal pain and diarrhea due to cold, certain chronic diseases like asthma and pulmonary tuberculosis.

五、禁忌证

对颜面、五官、大血管处不宜用直接灸；孕妇的腹部、腰骶部不宜施灸。

Ⅴ. Contraindication

It is inadvisable to perform direct moxibustion on the face, five sense organs, or the regions with major vessels. The abdominal region and lumbosacral region of pregnant women should not be moxibusted.

第二节　技术操作
Section Two　Operation Techniques

一、器械材料准备

艾绒、姜片、毫针等。

Ⅰ. Materials

Moxa, ginger slices, needles.

二、操作步骤

1. 无瘢痕灸

艾柱直接放置在皮肤上，点燃让其燃烧。当艾柱燃剩至 2/5，病人感到灼痛时，立即更换艾柱再灸，灸至局部皮肤发红而不起泡为度。

2. 瘢痕灸

在艾柱燃尽后才更换艾柱，直到燃完规定壮数为止。灸至局部皮肤起泡，灸后 1 周左右局部化脓，5—6 周后自行痊愈，结痂脱落，留有瘢痕。

3. 间接灸

将新鲜生姜或大蒜切成 0.2—0.3 厘米的薄片，并在其中间用针刺数孔，置于施术部位，上置艾柱施灸。待艾柱燃尽后，更换艾柱再灸。灸至局部皮肤发红而不起泡为度。

4. 艾条灸

将艾条的一段点燃，对准施灸部位熏烤，距离皮肤约 3 厘米，或作上下，左右，回旋等方式的移动，以病人有热感而无灼痛为宜。

5. 温针灸

在针刺留针时，将一团艾绒捏在针柄上，或截下一段长约 2 厘米的艾条插套在针柄上点燃，待燃尽后除去灰烬，再出针。

Ⅱ. Procedures

1. Non-scarring Moxibustion

When the 2/5 of a moxa cone is burnt, or when the patient feels a burning pain, replace another moxa cone. The moxibustion continues until the local skin becomes reddish but not blistered.

2. Scarring Moxibustion

Replace a new moxa cone until the previous one is burnt out. This procedure continues until the blisters are formed. About one week after moxibustion, suppuration is formed at the local region. And about 5 – 6 weeks later, the wound heals and the scab and scar is formed.

3. Indirect Moxibustion

A slice of fresh ginger or garlic about 0.2 – 0.3 cm thick is placed on the selected acupoint, with holes punched on that. A moxa cone is placed on the ginger slice and ignited. When it is burnt out, replace another one. This procedure continues until the local skin turns reddish but not blistered.

4. Moxibustion with Moxa Roll

An ignited moxa roll is pointed 3 cm above the region and moved upward and downward, to the left and right or get round. The patient feels warm but not scorching.

5. Moxibustion with Warmed Needle

During the retention of acupuncture, the needle handle is wrapped with some moxa or coated with one section of a moxa roll about 2 cm in length to be burnt. The needle is withdrawn after the moxa completely burns out and the ash is cleared.

三、治疗时间及疗程

根据患者的体质、年龄、施灸部位、所患病情等方面，每次施灸的量和疗程都是不同的。

临床上施灸的量，是以艾柱的大小和壮数的多少来计算的。艾柱分为大中小三种。青壮年男性、新病、体实者，宜大柱多壮；妇女、儿童、老人、久病、体弱者，宜小柱少壮。头面、四肢、皮薄肌少处，宜小柱少壮；腰腹、皮厚肉深处，不妨大柱多状。

施灸疗程的长短，可根据病情灵活掌握。急性病疗程较短，有时只需艾灸治疗 1—2 次即可；慢性病疗程较长，可灸数月乃至 1 年以上。一般初灸时，每日 1 次，3 日后改为 2—3 天1 次。

Ⅲ. Duration and Course of Treatment

The duration and course of moxibustion differs based on the constitution, age, the part needed to be moxibusted and the disease conditions.

One small pyramid-shaped piles of moxa is known as Zhu (cone) in Chinese. A cone after it has been burned is called one Zhuang. Therefore, Zhu and Zhuang are used for counting. The size of the moxa cone can be classified into large cone, medium cone, and small cone. For a person who is comparatively healthy and is in the beginning stage of a disease, one should use a large moxa cone for many Zhuangs, whereas a person who is less healthy and has a chronic illness should be treated with small cones for fewer Zhuangs. When using moxa on the head, face, fingers and chest area, the moxa cones should be small with fewer Zhuangs. When treating the back and stomach area, larger cones and more applications can be used.

It may takes once or twice moxibustion for some acute diseases, whereas several months or more than one year for some chronic diseases. At the beginning of the course, moxibust once for a day, and then slows down to once every 2 to 3 days after 3-days' treatment.

四、关键技术环节

(1) 施术者应严肃认真,向患者说明施术要求,消除其恐惧心理。如选用瘢痕灸时,必须先征得患者同意。

(2) 施灸时,患者应选择正确的体位。要求患者的体位宜平正舒适,有利于准确定穴,又利于艾柱的安放和施灸的顺利完成。

(3) 结合患者实际情况,选择艾柱的大小和灸壮的多少。

Ⅳ. Key Techniques

(1) The operator should take it seriously to explain the requirements to the patient in order to release his/her fear. Consent should be given by patient while the scar moxibustion is applied.

(2) The patient should take a appropriate posture, so the acupoints can be located well, the moxa cones can be placed well and the procedure will be done smoothly as well.

(3) Choosing the proper size of moxa cone and the quantity of Zhuangs according to the severity of disease.

五、注意事项

对颜面、五官、大血管处不宜用直接灸;孕妇的腹部、腰骶部不宜施灸。对肢体麻木不仁、感觉迟钝者,应注意勿灸过量,以免烫伤。

Ⅴ. Notes

Direct moxibustion is inadvisable to perform on the face, five sense organs, or the regions with major vessels. The abdominal region and lumbosacral region of pregnant women should not be moxibusted. For the patients with numbness of limbs or bradyesthesia, moxibustion should be carefully applied to avoid burning.

六、可能的意外情况及处理方案

在施灸或温针灸时,要防止艾火脱落,以免造成皮肤和衣物的烧损。施灸过程中,要随时了解患者的反应,及时调整灸火与皮肤间的距离,以免造成烫伤。

Ⅵ. Possible Accidents and Management

Prevent the spark and ashes of burning moxa from falling on the skin or clothes during the moxibustion. Get to know the patients' reaction and adjust the space between moxa and skin to avoid burning.

第十二章　刮痧技术
Chapter Twelve　Skin Scraping

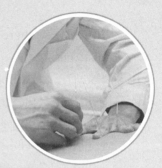

第一节　概　述
Section One　General Introduction

一、概念

刮痧是传统的自然疗法之一，用刮痧器具等刮拭经络、穴位等处，通过刺激使皮肤出现潮红、紫红或紫黑色的瘀斑，以改善局部微循环，起到扶正祛邪、疏通经络、祛风散寒等作用，从而达到防治疾病、养生保健等目的的一种疗法。

Ⅰ. Definition

As one of the traditional natural therapies, skin scraping refers to scrap meridians and acupoints with scraping tools. By stimulating, the skin becomes flush, purple or dark purple, which can improve local micro-circulation, reinforce healthy qi and expel pathogenic factors, dredge the meridians, expel wind and cold and so on, so as to prevent and treat disease, as well as health care.

二、治疗原理

刮痧疗法以中医皮部理论为基础，皮部，是经脉功能活动反应于体表的部位，也是络脉之气散布之所。皮部居人体的最外层，是机体的卫外屏障，机体卫外功能失调，外邪则通过皮肤深入络脉、经脉以及脏腑，引起疾病。另外机体内脏有病也可通过经脉络脉而反应于皮部。因此，刮痧通过刺激皮肤表面，可通过络脉、经脉深入脏腑而治疗疾病。

Ⅱ. Rationale of Treatment

Skin scraping therapy is based on Chinese medicine sheath theory. The sheath is the place where reflects functional activities of meridians, but also the region distributing the qi of the collaterals. Covering over the body, the sheath protects the body from pathogenic factors. When defensive functions are disordered, exogenous evils enter the collaterals, meridians and organs and cause diseases. Besides, when internal organs get sick, it can be reflected on the sheath through meridians and collaterals. Therefore, by stimulating the skin, skin scraping can treat disease through collaterals, meridians and organs in depth.

三、分类

按照是否使用刮痧工具,可以分为刮痧法与撮痧法。

1. 刮痧法

最常用的一种方法。刮痧部位通常在背部或颈部两侧,根据病情需要,有时也可在颈前喉头两侧,脊柱两侧,臂弯两侧或膝弯内侧等处。通常采用光滑的硬币、铜勺柄、瓷碗、药匙或特制的刮板,蘸取刮痧介质(如刮痧油、冷开水等),在体表特定部位反复刮动、摩擦。

2. 撮痧法

在患者的待刮拭部位涂上刮痧介质,然后施术者五指屈曲,将中指和食指等弯曲如钩状,蘸刮痧介质后夹揪或提扯皮肤,把皮肤和肌肉夹起然后用力向外滑动再松开,一夹一放,反复进行,并连续发出"巴巴"的声响。在同一部位可连续操作6—7遍,被夹起的部位就会出现痧痕,造成局部瘀血,使皮肤出现血痕的除痧方法。

Ⅲ. Classification

It can be classified to regular scraping and nipping scraping according to whether the scraping tools are used.

1. Regular Scraping

In this procedure, a lubricating medium, such as massage oil, is applied to the skin of the area to be treated. A smooth-edged instrument is used by the operator to apply on the skin, typically in the area of pain or on the back parallel to the spine, neck, throat, arm, and popliteal fossa as well.

2. Nipping Scraping

Before the process, the areas and fingers are moistened with water or oil, then use two fingers (the index and middle finger) to nip the skin forcefully and repeatedly. Nip for about 6 - 7 times in each region, until ellipse-shaped patch appears on the skin.

四、适应证

刮痧疗法是中医外治法之一,不仅可用于内科、儿科、骨伤科、五官科等各科疾病的治疗,而且可用于疾病的预防。对保健强身、美容美体、减肥也有明显的作用。

Ⅳ. Indications

Skin scraping is one of the TCM external therapies. It can be used in treatment of internal medicine, pediatrics, orthopedics, ENT, and the prevention of several diseases as well. It has good effects on health care, beauty and weight losing.

五、禁忌证

(1) 各类急慢性感染性疾病,如高热、急性骨髓炎、结核、感染性皮肤疾病、糖尿病及各类出血倾向疾病,如白血病和凝血功能障碍。

(2) 皮肤有溃疡、疮疡、烫伤、骨折或伤口等。

(3) 月经期或孕期妇女的腰骶部禁止刮痧。

(4) 过饥、过饱、极度劳累或紧张者,禁止刮痧。

Ⅴ. Contraindication

(1) It isn't allowed for those with various acute or chronic infectious diseases, such as fever, acute osteomyelitis, tuberculosis, contagious skin diseases, diabetes, and hemorrhagic conditions like thrombopenia or coagulation disorders.

(2) Body parts with skin ulcers, sores, scalding, recent fracture, or wounds cannot be scraped.

(3) Lumbosacral area of women during menstruation or pregnancy cannot be scraped.

(4) Those with excessive hunger, overeat, fatigue or nervousness are forbidden for skin scraping.

第二节　技术操作
Section Two　Operation Techniques

一、器械材料准备

刮痧器具:常用玉石和水牛角。

刮痧介质:常用有两大类。

(1) 液体为最常用的一种刮痧介质,最简单的可用我们日常生活中的饮用水(冷开水或温开水)、食用油、各种外涂药液等。

(2) 膏体质地细腻膏状的凡士林、面霜等、不同功效的药膏,如活血润肤膏、通络止痛膏、解毒膏等。

Ⅰ. Materials

Scraping tools: (commonly used) jade, horn.

Scraping medium:

(1) Liquid: Liquid is the most common scraping medium, such as drinking water (cold or warm), oil and medicinal liquid etc.

(2) Balm: Fine vaseline, lotion and certain medicinal balm, such as the balm of invigorating blood and moistening skin, the balm of dredging collaterals and relieving pain, the balm of resolving toxins.

二、操作步骤

（1）先暴露患者的刮痧部位，用干净毛巾蘸肥皂，将此部位洗擦干净。

（2）手法：施术者用右手拿取操作工具，蘸植物油或清水后，在确定的体表部位，轻轻向下顺刮或从内向外反复刮动，逐渐加重，刮时要沿同一方向刮，力量要均匀，采用腕力，一般刮 10—20 次，以出现紫红色斑点或斑块为度。

（3）一般要求先刮颈项部，再刮脊椎两侧部，然后再刮胸部及四肢部位。

Ⅱ. Procedures

(1) The area to be scraped is first exploded and cleaned by soap.

(2) Manipulations: The operator rubs with an instrument lubricated with oil or water in downward strokes. Once the area is localized, scrap the area from up to down or from the internal to the external repeatedly. The strengths need to be even. The doctor should scrap the area with the strengths of the wrist. Generally speaking, the area needs to be scrapped for 10 to 20 times until the petechiae are completely raised.

(3) From the neck to the lateral side of spine, and from the chest to limbs.

三、治疗时间及疗程

每个治疗部位一般刮 10—20 次，以出现紫红色斑点或斑块为度。一般两次刮痧间隔3—5 天，但具体要看前一次痧痕是否退尽，即以痧痕是否退尽决定下次刮治时间。以 5—6 次为一个疗程。

Ⅲ. Duration and Course of Treatment

Generally speaking, every area can be scraped 10 - 20 times, until the petechiae are completely raised. After 3 - 5 days, the second scraping can be continued if the petechiae vanishes. It takes $5-6$ times treatment for one course.

四、关键技术环节

1. 辨证明确是提高刮痧疗效的基础

辨证施治是中医治疗学的核心,刮痧疗法也不例外。对于任何一种疾病首先要辨明阴阳、表里、寒热、虚实,根据其偏盛偏衰采取不同的补泻手法,虚者补之,实则泻之。

2. 经穴准确是提高刮痧疗效的关键

刮痧疗法以经络理论为基础,因此辨证明确后选经取穴是关键,根据疾病的病因、病位、病性及标本缓急选经取穴。遵循"宁失一穴,不失一经"的原则,熟练掌握经络的循行规律和经穴的部位,循经刮痧既有点又有线还有面,经脉穴位尽在其中。

3. 手法正确是提高刮痧疗效的重点

刮痧经穴确定后手法至关重要,根据病人的年龄、体质、虚实施以正确的补泻手法才能调整脏腑、阴阳、气血经络虚实,使之平衡,若手法不明,补泻不清,则难以提高疗效。

Ⅳ. Key Techniques

1. Right Differentiation is the Basis of Effects of Scrapping

Syndrome differentiation is the core of TCM, so is the scraping therapy. For any disease, we must first identify the yin and yang, exterior and interior, cold and heat, the deficiency and excess, then take a different approach based on reinforcing and reducing situation.

2. The Accuracy of Acupoints is the Key of Scraping Effects

Scraping therapy is based on meridian theory, so after the syndrome differentiation, it is essential to select acupoints according to the cause of the disease, disease location, disease property and priorities. Follow the principle of "losing an acupoint is preferred to losing a meridian"; master the law of meridian routine and the site of acupoints. The place to be scraped includes acupoints, meridians and even area.

3. The Correct Technique is the Focus of Efficacy of Scrapping

Scraping technique is essential after the acupoints are selected. According to the patient's age, constitution, excess or deficiency, implement the right reinforcing and reducing method to adjust the internal organs, yin and yang, qi and blood, meridians and collaterals, excess and deficiency for balance. If the technique is unknown, and reinforcing and reducing is unclear, the effects of scrapping is difficult to improve.

五、注意事项

(1) 实施刮痧治疗时,室内要安静、清洁、通风,室温要适中。

(2) 刮拭前要向患者介绍刮痧常识,可能出现的情况,以取得患者的配合。

（3）刮痧前要对患者刮拭部位常规消毒，施刮者双手也要消毒，刮痧板最好一人一板，以免交叉感染，刮痧板每次用完后要消毒，并妥善保管。

（4）不可在过饥、过饱、过度紧张、过度疲劳或酒后刮治以免发生晕刮。

（5）不可强求出痧。

（6）刮痧治疗后要饮水，补充消耗的水分。

（7）刮痧治疗后为避免外邪侵袭，须在皮肤毛孔闭合恢复原状后方可洗浴，一般 2—3 小时。

Ⅴ. Notes

（1）The clinic should be quiet, clean and well ventilated; temperature should be moderate.

（2）Introduce the whole procedure to the patient before it is started.

（3）Routine disinfection of the treating area should be done before scraping, as well as the operator's hands, and the scraping plates. It is preferable that one plate is only for one patient, so as to avoid cross-infection. Scraping plates should be disinfected after using and keep it properly.

（4）Patients with excessive hunger, excessive intake, fatigue, nervousness or drinking should avoid scraping.

（5）The red or purple petechiae cannot be forced out.

（6）Drinking water after scraping.

（7）After scraping, avoid the attack of exogenous evils. Therefore, bath after the pores close. Generally, it takes about 2 - 3 hours.

六、可能的意外情况及处理方案

刮痧疗法和针灸一样，有可能像晕针一样出现晕刮。晕刮的症状为头晕，面色苍白、心慌、出冷汗、四肢发冷，恶心欲吐或神昏扑倒等。

1. 预防措施

空腹、过度疲劳患者忌刮；低血压、低血糖、过度虚弱和神经紧张特别怕痛的患者轻刮。

2. 急救措施

迅速让患者平卧；让患者饮用 1 杯温糖开水。

Ⅵ. Possible Accident and Processing

Like acupuncture, faint scraping might appear. It is characterized by dizziness, pale complexion, fluster, sweating, cold limbs, nausea with desire to spit or faint, etc.

1. Prevention Measures

Hungry, excessively tired patients should avoid scraping; those with low blood pressure, low blood sugar, excessive weakness, nervousness and fear of pain should be scraped mildly.

2. Emergency Measures

Let patients lie down quickly; drink 1 cup of warm sugar water.

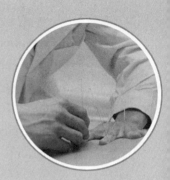

第十三章　拔罐技术
Chapter Thirteen　Cupping

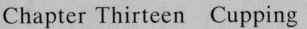

第一节　概　述
Section One　General Introduction

一、概念

拔罐是以罐杯为工具，用燃烧等方法造成罐内负压而吸附于皮肤上，引起局部充血从而达到一定防治疾病效果的一种方法。大多数拔罐是用火来操作产生吸力的，因此常常叫作"火罐"。

Ⅰ. Definition

Cupping is a therapy in which a jar is attached to the skin surface by introducing a flame into the cup or some other means that create negative pressure for suction. By forming a localized congestion, diseases can be prevented or treated. Most cupping done in ancient times is flame-induced suction, hence the name "Flame cupping" is commonly used.

二、治疗原理

拔罐疗法也是以中医理论为基础，认为拔罐可以疏通经络之气血，调节脏腑之功能，从而达到治病的目的。也可以理解成，拔罐的负压可以形成吸力，导致局部地充血，把病理产物通过肌肤腠理从体内排出。

Ⅱ. Rationale of Treatment

Cupping therapy is based on Chinese medicine theory. Cupping is able to dredge the meridians' qi and blood, and adjust organs function to achieve the purpose of curing the diseases. The vacuum has a strong pull of the suction force on the meridian points, then the skin becomes reddish and congestive so that the body's pathological product can be removed out of the body from the skin pores.

三、分类

1. 留罐

拔罐后,留置一定的时间,一般留置 5—15 分钟。这种方法用于很多种疾病,可以单个或者多个罐一起拔。

2. 闪罐

罐子拔上后,立即起下,反复吸拔多次,至皮肤潮红、充血为止。多用于不能耐受留罐的患者如小孩,或者脸部的一些病证。

3. 推罐

又称走罐,最好用玻璃罐,先在罐口涂一些润滑油脂,将罐吸上后,以手握住罐底,慢慢向前推动,这样在皮肤表面上下或左右来回推拉移动数次,至皮肤潮红为止。一般用于面积较大,肌肉丰富的部位,如腰背、大腿等部。

4. 针罐

先在一定的部位施行针刺,待达到一定的刺激量后,将针留在原处,再以针刺处为中心,拔上火罐 5—10 分钟,直至局部充血潮红后起罐。这种方法结合了针刺和拔罐两种疗法的作用。

5. 刺血拔罐

局部仔细消毒后,用三棱针等,根据按病变部位的大小和出血要求,按刺血法刺破小血管,然后拔以火罐,留罐 5—10 分钟。可以加强刺血法的效果,常用于一些急性扭伤、丹毒等急症。

Ⅲ. Classification

1. Retaining Cupping

Attach the cup to the skin and retain it for 5 to 10 minutes, and remove it. This is used for many disorders. In clinical practice, a single-cup or multi-cup retaining can be used.

2. Flashing Cupping

Attach and remove the cup quickly and repeatedly until the treated area becomes reddish, congested or extravagated. This is used on patients who cannot accept retaining cupping such as infants, or for treatments done on the face.

3. Sliding Cupping

Spread some vaseline or paraffin oil to the treated area; attach the cup to the skin; move it up and down or left and right on the selected area, and finally remove the cup when the skin becomes reddish and congestive. This method is suitable for places with thick muscles in large areas, such as waist, back and thighs.

4. Needling-retaining Cupping

This method is a combination of acupuncture and cupping. Attach a cup to the area around one or more of the retained needles and keep the needles inside the cup. Remove the cup and needles after 5 to 10 minutes, or when the localized skin becomes reddish, congested or extravagated.

5. Blood-letting and Cupping

Carefully disinfect the area to be treated. Prick the points with a three-edged needle to induce bleeding, and then attach the cup to the appropriate points. Retain the cup on the area for 5 to 10 minutes. This is a way to strengthen the effects of the blood-letting. It is indicated for erysipelas, sprains and acute mastitis.

四、适应证

拔罐适应证较广，例如风寒湿痹证、急性扭伤、感冒、哮喘、消化不良、胃痛等等。此外，该法还可以治疗一些外科病证，如丹毒、蛇虫咬伤等。

Ⅳ. Indications

Cupping has numerous indications, such as arthritis due to wind-cold-dampness, acute sprains, common cold, cough, asthma, indigestion, stomachache etc. In addition, this therapy can treat some surgical diseases such as erysipelas and snake bite.

五、禁忌证

拔罐通常不在骨骼凸出或者毛发浓密的部位进行操作。

拔罐不可在溃疡、水肿和过敏的部位操作，不可在大血管分布的部位，孕妇的腰骶和腹部，以及高热、抽搐的病人。

Ⅴ. Contraindication

Cupping should be applied to areas with thick muscles rather than the bony and hairy areas.

It is ill-advised to apply cupping to areas containing an allergic reaction, ulcers and edema; to places where large vessels are distributed, to the abdomen, waist and sacrum of pregnant women, and to patients with spasms and a higher fever.

第二节　技术操作
Section Two　Operation Techniques

一、拔罐器具的准备

根据需要选择合适的罐杯,有玻璃罐、竹罐、陶罐以及抽气罐等。

Ⅰ. Preparation of Cupping Tools

Choose the suitable cup. There are glass cup, bamboo cup, pottery jar, piston air-sucking cup.

二、操作步骤

用镊子夹住一个 95% 的乙醇棉球,点燃后在罐内绕 1—2 圈即退出,迅速将火罐扣在施术部位,称为闪罐法。一般留置 5—10 分钟。起罐时;以食指在罐口旁的皮肤上略加按压,使空气进入罐内,便可取下火罐。

Ⅱ. Procedures

Ignite a 95% alcohol-soaked cotton ball held with tweezers, put the flame into the cup and circle the flame inside it for 1 to 2 times. Remove the flame and place the cup onto the skin very quickly. The cups could be retained on the skin for 5 - 10 minutes. The attached cup should be removed by holding it with the left hand and pressing the skin around the cup with the thumb or index finger of the right hand to let air in. Don't remove the cup by force.

三、治疗时间及疗程

根据病人情况,每次拔罐 5—10 分钟不等。一般两次拔罐间隔 5—7 天,具体要看前一次拔罐的罐印是否退尽,即以罐印是否退尽决定下次拔罐时间。以 5—6 次为一个疗程。

Ⅲ. Duration and Course of Treatment

Generally speaking, cupping lasts for 5 - 10 minutes based on the patients' condition. After 5 - 7 days, the second cupping treatment can be continued if the cupping print vanished. That's to say, whether the cupping print is completely disappeared is the evidence for the next cupping. It takes 5 - 6 times' treatment for one course.

四、关键技术环节

1. 辨证明确是提高拔罐疗效的基础

辨证施治是中医治疗学的核心，拔罐疗法也不例外。对于任何一种疾病首先要辨明阴阳、表里、寒热、虚实，根据其偏盛偏衰采取不同的补泻手法，虚者补之，实则泻之。

2. 经穴准确是提高拔罐疗效的关键

拔罐疗法以经络理论为基础，因此辨证明确后选经取穴是关键，根据疾病的病因、病位、病性以及标本缓急选经取穴。

Ⅳ. Key Techniques

1. Right Differentiation is the Basis of Effects of Cupping

Syndrome differentiation is the core of TCM, so is the Cupping therapy. For any disease, we must first identify the yin and yang, exterior and interior, cold and heat, the deficiency and excess, and then take a different approach, reinforcing or reducing. Reinforce the deficiency and reduce the excess.

2. The Accuracy of Acupoints is the Key of Cupping Effect

Cupping therapy is based on meridian theory, so after the syndrome differentiation, it is very important to select acupoints according to the cause of the disease, disease location, disease property and priorities.

五、注意事项

（1）实施拔罐治疗时，室内要安静、清洁、通风，室温要适中。

（2）根据拔罐部位，选择大小合适的罐杯。拔罐前要向患者介绍拔罐常识，可能出现的情况，以取得患者的配合。

（3）拔罐前要对患者相应部位及术者双手常规消毒，罐用过后要注意消毒，以免发生交叉感染，并放好罐具。

（4）拔罐的过程必须非常细心。不可在过饥、过饱、过度紧张、过度疲劳或酒后拔罐以免发生晕罐。

（5）拔罐治疗后要饮水，补充消耗的水分。

（6）拔罐治疗后为避免外邪侵袭，须在皮肤毛孔闭合恢复原状后方可洗浴，一般 2—3 小时。

Ⅴ. Notes

（1）The clinic should be quiet, clean and well ventilated. Temperature should be moderate.

(2) Select the proper sized cups depending on the areas to be treated. Introduce the whole procedure to the patient before it is started.

(3) Before cupping, disinfect the area to be treated and the operator's hands to avoid cross-infection. Cups should be disinfected after using and keep them properly.

(4) The cupping procedure should be done with great care. Patients with excessive hunger, excessive intake, nervousness or fatigue should avoid cupping.

(5) Drink some warm water after cupping to supplement the consumed water.

(6) After cupping, avoid the attack of exogenous evils. Therefore, bath after the pores close. Generally, it takes about 2 – 3 hours.

六、可能的意外情况及处理方案

拔罐疗法和针灸一样,有可能像晕针一样出现晕罐。晕罐的症状为头晕,面色苍白、心慌、出冷汗、四肢发冷,恶心欲吐或神昏扑倒等。

1. 预防措施

空腹、过度疲劳患者忌刮;低血压、低血糖、过度虚弱和神经紧张特别怕痛的患者罐要少,吸力要轻。

2. 急救措施

迅速让患者平卧;让患者饮用 1 杯温糖开水。

Ⅵ. Possible Accident and Processing

Like acupuncture, cupping might lead to fainting. There are symptoms like dizziness, pale complexion, fluster, sweating, cold limbs, nausea to vomit or faint, etc.

1. Prevention Measures

Hungry and tired patients should avoid cupping; for those with low blood pressure, low blood sugar, excessive weakness, nervousness and fear of pain, we should use less cups and mild forces.

2. Emergency Measures

Let patients lie down quickly and drink a cup of warm sugar water.

参考文献
References

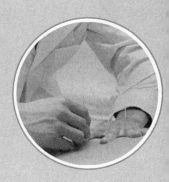

［1］马淑然,刘兴仁.中医基础理论(汉英对照)［M］.北京：中国中医药出版社,2015.

［2］柴可夫.中医基础理论［M］.2版.北京：人民卫生出版社,1998.

［3］胡冬裴.中医基础理论：数字化中英文教材 The Basic Theory of Chinese Medicine：Digital Chinese-English Text Book(配光盘)［M］.北京：清华大学出版社,2013.

［4］左言富.新编实用中医文库：中医基础理论(英汉对照)［M］.上海：上海浦江教育出版社有限公司,2003.

［5］印会河.中医基础理论［M］.上海：上海科学技术出版社,1984.

［6］俞大方.推拿学.上海：上海科学技术出版社,1985.

［7］丁季峰.中国医学百科全书·推拿学［M］.上海：上海科学技术出版社,1987.

［8］曹仁发.中医推拿学［M］.北京：人民卫生出版社,1992.

［9］严隽陶.推拿学［M］.北京：中国中医药出版社,2009.

［10］房敏.推拿学［M］.北京：人民卫生出版社,2012.

［11］王之虹.推拿学［M］.北京：高等教育出版社,2013.

［12］王之虹.推拿手法学［M］.北京：人民卫生出版社,2016.

［13］范炳华.推拿治疗学［M］.北京：中国中医药出版社,2016.

［14］房敏,宋柏林.推拿学［M］.北京：中国中医药出版社,2016.

［15］刘明军,王金贵.小儿推拿学［M］.北京：中国中医药出版社,2016.

［16］赵京生,左言富,李照国.中国针灸(英汉对照)［M］.上海：上海浦江教育出版社,2002.

［17］王文秀,贾轶群,王颖.英汉对照中医英语会话［M］.北京：人民卫生出版社,2014.

［18］李照国,张庆荣.中医英语(附光盘)［M］.2版.上海：上海科学技术出版社,2013.